• IN SEARCH OF SAFETY

IN SEARCH OF SAFETY

• CHEMICALS AND CANCER RISK •

John D. Graham, Laura C. Green,
and Marc J. Roberts

HARVARD UNIVERSITY PRESS
Cambridge, Massachusetts, and London, England   1988

Library of Congress Cataloging-in-Publication Data

Graham, John D. (John David), 1956–
   In search of safety.

   Bibliography: p.
   Includes index.
   1. Carcinogens—Safety regulations—United States.
2. Carcinogens—Government policy—United States.
3. Benzene—Health aspects. 4. Formaldehyde—Health
aspects. I. Green, Laura C. II. Roberts, Marc J.
III. Title.
RC268.6.G73 1988   363.1'79   88-11011
ISBN 0-674-44635-6 (alk. paper)

▪ CONTENTS

FOREWORD

by Harvey Brooks

PUBLIC POLICY in all industrialized countries is increasingly challenged by issues in which scientific and technological considerations are paramount. Especially in the United States, policy makers and the public continue to hope that more research and "better science" will lead to greater consensus on the "facts" and thereby help resolve policy questions. Enormous effort and thought go into the creation of mechanisms for improving the quality of the scientific information used in making such policy decisions.

Good science would certainly help resolve science-intensive policy decisions in the long run, but administrative, legislative, and judical processes are seldom permitted that much time. A growing body of experience seems to suggest that, in fact, more research and better technical information actually exacerbate conflict among experts and in the policy process. This situation is especially well documented in the case of regulatory policy for toxic chemicals. How can this be true, and what does it mean? Why does more and better information seem only to raise more questions than it answers and increase both the disagreement among the experts and the polarization of the public policy debate?

Some commentators have even proposed seriously that we ignore the experts and follow popular instincts; they suggest that science simply confuses democratic decision making and that the call for better science is simply a delaying tactic on the part of regulated industries and other groups that prefer the status quo.

There is an enormous literature on this question, particularly as it pertains to environmental regulation. The authors of this book approach the general issue by looking at the attempts to regulate two specific suspected carcinogens, benzene and formaldehyde, from several different perspectives. They examine in great detail the scientific evidence bearing on the risks of public exposure to these chemicals, and they describe some of the processes that have been tried to resolve disagreement among experts concerning the magnitude of these risks. They analyze the political and judicial responses to technical disagreement, carefully describing the reaction of numerous people, both scientists and nonscientists, to each new scientific finding, sketching the growing complexity and confusion of the technical and the legal-political situation as knowledge supposedly improves.

The authors' most important conclusion is that the problem they describe so clearly is the result in part of excessive and unrealistic expectations of science—not in its ultimate aspirations but in its current state of development as related to the information needs of regulators. We tend to exaggerate what we really know through science unless we are challenged by the social consequences of the findings. When the interpretation of scientific findings has large distributional consequences for different groups—health risks for some and economic dislocation for others, for example—we become more aware of the large uncertainties in our knowledge and of the inadequacies of our theories and models. According to the authors, the first instinct of the scientists is to close ranks and produce a consensus that papers over their disagreements and the underlying uncertainties. This course of action is powerfully reinforced by regulators who need seemingly objective information to defend the decisions they must make—decisions that will be challenged in court if they cannot be justified "scientifically." Yet, to the extent that the scientists suppress uncertainties, they are in effect arrogating to themselves a political decision for which they are not accountable, since each choice of information within a wide band of uncertainty creates different winners and losers and hence is inherently political. In other words, an artificial consensus among scientists is undemocratic in its implications. Only if they are completely honest about the extent of their ignorance are they playing a role appropriate to democratic polity.

The authors see no way out of this dilemma except to recommend that scientific advisory groups be completely open about their lack of consensus and the scientific reasons for it, forcing politically accountable officials to make the choices which only they can properly make in a representative government. They do offer some hope that as scientists discover more of the causal mechanisms underlying the health effects of chemicals—including the routes of exposure as well as the biological mechanisms at the cellular and molecular levels—

they will be able to make quantitative risk assessments with the reliability that the legal-political system pretends is possible today. But that happy time may be a long way off, and no one can predict when it will arrive.

The "maturing" of a branch of science usually entails progress from statistical description to the elucidation of causal mechanisms or models which permit more reliable extrapolation from situations in which association of antecedents and effects is readily measurable to those less amenable to measurement or experiment. It would be interesting to study other cases in which policy decisions hinged on scientific conclusions where causal chains were more completely understood. One might thereby find a relationship between the "maturity" of a branch of science and its appropriate role in public policy decisions. I suspect that as a branch of science becomes truly mature public policy decisions which hinge on it will gradually cease to be controversial.

Some readers will undoubtedly feel that this conclusion is a counsel of perfection, that the buck will not be passed from scientists to regulators because the scientists who are attracted to the regulatory system enjoy the feeling of power it confers on them, while the regulators and politicians are only too happy to leave the decisions to "science." The danger, say the authors, is that the public will lose confidence in science and will withdraw its support for the research required to progress from the feeble and expensive statistical risk assessment techniques available today to a truly causal theory of carcinogenesis and other health effects.

Although the particular examples of benzene and formaldehyde are highly special, I believe that many of the lessons presented here will apply much more broadly to the question of scientific advice in the policy process. I also hope that the work the authors have done will open up an important new field of research from which we will be able to learn which features of these cases are peculiar to that particular area of science and which aspects are truly generalizable.

• PREFACE

THIS BOOK is about the controversies that arise in the regulation of chemicals that are known or suspected to cause cancer. The book attempts to dissect and illuminate the controversies through an intellectual approach we call "scientific conflict mapping." We conclude with some recommendations designed to clarify and strengthen the important yet limited role that science can play in the resolution of these disputes.

The book is the final product of the Scientific Conflict Mapping Project (1983–1986), Department of Health Policy and Management, Harvard School of Public Health. The project had its origins in a letter to Harvard President Derek Bok from James Mathis, Vice President for Research of the Exxon Corporation. Mathis was interested in exploring how the university could work cooperatively with industry and other segments of society to develop better ways to resolve the scientific conflicts that arise in the course of chemical regulation. President Bok passed Mathis's letter along to Dean Howard Hiatt of the School of Public Health. Hiatt enlisted Marc J. Roberts, who, drawing on some of his earlier work, led the effort to develop the intellectual design and work plan for what ultimately became the Scientific Conflict Mapping Project.

Initially the project was funded by a mixture of corporate and foundation support, most notably a grant from the Alfred P. Sloan Foundation and a grant from a consortium of six corporations (Dow Chemical Company, E. I. duPont de Nemours and Company, Exxon Corporation, Mobil Research and Development Corporation, Monsanto Company, and Rohm and Haas Company). In its later stages, the project was also supported by U.S. Environmental Protection Agency Assistance Agreement CR807809 to Interdisciplinary Programs in Health (Harvard School of Public Health) and institutional resources of the School of Public Health. It is with deep gratitude that we acknowledge and thank each of our sponsors and the support of Deans Howard Hiatt and Harvey Fineberg of the School of Public Health.

The plan for the project was developed with the guidance of a distinguished steering committee: Harvey Brooks, Douglas Costle, Howard Hiatt, Cyrus Levinthal, James Mathis, Dorothy Nelkin, Howard Raiffa, Ellen Silbergeld, and Monte Throdahl. We thank each of them for their ideas, their generous commitments of time, and their patience.

In the course of the project we sponsored three meetings in Boston to explore the sources of scientific disagreement. We learned a great deal from these meetings about our case studies—benzene and formaldehyde—as well as about procedural considerations in the elicitation of scientific judgments. We thank all the eager and thoughtful participants in the meetings (they are listed individually in the Appendix).

Toward the end of the project, we asked our colleagues to help us sharpen our message, correct errors, and polish the manuscript. The responses were extremely useful. In particular we thank John Bailar, Evelyn Brodkin, Harvey Brooks, John Evans, Adam Finkel, John Harrison, Dale Hattis, Henry Heck, Donald Hornig, William Lowrance, John McCullough, John Mendeloff, Frederick Mosteller, Dorothy Nelkin, Catherine Petito, James Senger, Mary White, and James Wilson. Obviously, neither they nor the members of our steering committee agree with all we have said or bear any responsibility for our conclusion.

Finally, and most important, we acknowledge the tireless efforts of all those who worked with us. Michael Dowling, the first employee of the project, helped get it started. Stephen Thomas, who was for a time co-principal investigator, assisted us throughout both intellectually and administratively. With Marc Roberts, he was a co-author of a paper on conflict mapping that the project produced. Laura Green served as director of scientific research for the project. John Graham joined as a postdoctoral fellow and served as co-principal investigator in the later stages. Angela Boggs provided important research assistance, played the key role in organizing our meetings, and generally made things happen. Scott Wolff wrote the memorandum that led to our selection of benzene and formaldehyde as case studies. Ms. Boggs and Mr. Wolff deserve special recognition for their help in preparing early drafts of several chapters. Word processing was competently done by Carol Perez, Elaine Rossignol, Jenny Taylor, and Rebecca Welch. Without all this help, we might not have started and certainly would not have finished.

In a book that reflects collaboration of individuals from different disciplines, the issue of responsibility for authorship inevitably arises. We have listed ourselves alphabetically to indicate our fully equal and collegial participation in and responsibility for the entire manuscript. Although each author brought different strengths and background to the task, we all contributed to, argued about, modified, edited, and shaped each chapter. Our goal has been to make the entire book accessible to an audience with a range of backgrounds. We hope that the reader will profit as much from our collaboration as we as individuals already have.

· ABBREVIATIONS

AAF   2-acetylaminofluorine
AIHC   American Industrial Health Council
AFL–CIO   American Federation of Labor—Council of Industrial Organizations
ALL   acute lymphyocytic leukemia
AML   acute myelogenous leukemia
ANLL   acute nonlymphocytic leukemia
ANSI   American National Standards Institute
API   American Petroleum Institute
APHA   American Public Health Association
BAT   best available technology
BCME   bischloromethyl ether
CAG   Carcinogen Assessment Group
CBA   cost-benefit analysis
CEA   cost-effectiveness analysis
CIIT   Chemical Industry Institute of Technology
CLL   chronic lymphocytic leukemia
CML   chronic myelogenous leukemia
CPSC   Consumer Products Safety Commission
DHS   Department of Health Services (California)
DNA   deoxyribonucleic acid
EDB   ethylene dibromide
EDF   Environmental Defense Fund
ETS   emergency temporary standard
ETU   ethylene thiourea
FI   Formaldehyde Institute
HCl   hydrochloric acid

IARC   International Agency for Research on Cancer
IRLG   Interagency Regulatory Liaison Group
MLE   maximum likelihood estimate
MNNG   methylnitronitrosoguanidine
MRC   Medical Research Council
NAS   National Academy of Sciences
NCTR   National Center for Toxicological Research
NIOSH   National Institute for Occupational Safety and Health
NOEL   no-observable-effects level
NRC   National Research Council
NRDC   National Resources Defense Council
NTP   National Toxicology Program
NYU   New York University
OMB   Office of Management and Budget
OSTP   Office of Science and Technology Policy
ORA   Office of Risk Assessment
OTS   Office of Toxic Substances
PEL   permissible exposure limit
ppb   parts per billion
ppm   parts per million
QRA   quantitative risk assessment
TSCA   Toxic Substances Control Act
TWA   time-weighted average
UAW   United Auto Workers
UCL   upper confidence limit
UFFI   urea formaldehyde foam insulation
URW   United Rubber Workers

▪ IN SEARCH OF SAFETY

1 ▪ OBJECTIVES AND METHODS

WE LIVE in a world rife with controversies about chemicals and human health. Claims and counterclaims are made to legislators, judges, and public officials about the dangers of exposure to substances such as arsenic, asbestos, benzene, formaldehyde, gasoline, polychlorinated biphenyls (PCBs), and radon. Typically, these controversies involve a very confused mixture of science and politics, including debates about what substances may present risks, what margins of safety are achievable and prudent, and what cleanup costs are necessary and affordable.[1]

Much of the concern has been about substances that may cause cancer, which is hardly surprising, given that one in three Americans develops cancer and one in four dies of it.[2] And there is a widespread belief that many human cancers are attributable to chemicals in our food and water, at our places of work, and even in our homes.[3] Public concern is magnified by the perception that some cancer risks are imposed upon workers, consumers, and citizens without their knowledge and with no means to control their exposures.[4]

The controversies about known and potential chemical carcinogens arise in part from differences in people's values and interests. To some, the mere possibility of an increase in cancer risk, no matter how small or speculative, is sufficient to justify severe regulatory restrictions on the use of a suspect chemical. Others argue that in light of the economic benefits many chemicals provide, we ought not to worry about such risks until they are convincingly proven to be substantial. Still others argue for various intermediary positions. And these different points of view receive support from organized interest groups such as environmental, health, and consumer advocacy groups, labor unions, and chemical manufacturers and users.

Although these differences in values and interests are important, the controversies are not solely political. Scientifically, the causes of cancer are only incompletely understood.[5] Ask a group of scientists about the magnitude of the cancer risk posed by formaldehyde, for example, and you may find each member of the group articulating quite a different view about how to interpret the available epidemiological data and how to extrapolate results from laboratory animal experiments to humans, about what theories of carcinogenesis are plausible and what research agendas are likely to be fruitful.

Ordinary citizens are accustomed to being bombarded with conflicting claims and counterclaims about controversial policy issues. But the frequent, heated, and often radical disagreements among apparently qualified scientists make the toxic chemical issue especially difficult for citizens—and for their nonexpert political representatives—to comprehend. The resulting confusion, it has been argued, endangers the health of both science and democracy.[6] The intermingling of scientific and political conflict tends to obscure the extent of technical knowledge and professional agreement. The resulting cynicism reinforces the (we believe incorrect) view that scientists do not really know anything and that they will sell their opinions to the highest bidder. When the public starts entertaining such views, responsible decision making can be undermined. If no one knows anything, and the respective roles of fact and value are obscure, regulators cannot possibly be held responsible either for their scientific errors or for their policy judgments.

• Objectives

In this book we investigate some controversies about regulating selected chemical carcinogens. Our first goal is to clarify the scientific and policy questions that are central to such regulatory decisions. We contrast the kinds of questions that regulators pose to scientists with the rather different kinds of questions that scientists ask of themselves.

Second, we seek to explain how and why scientists disagree about the answers to questions that are of importance to regulators. We find that scientists face profound challenges in trying to answer questions that are sometimes only partly scientific and that often transcend current knowledge of carcinogenesis.[7] In addition, genuine technical disagreements arise from differences in professional training, disciplinary orientation, and intellectual style—as well as from variations in personal intuition and judgment. And in some cases scientists, like other people, seem to act at least in part under the conscious or subconscious desire to influence policy results. (Such behavior does not necessarily reflect evil intentions; one scientist may feel an ethical obligation to counteract what he perceives as the clear errors or biases of a colleague.)

Our third, related goal is to present the promise as well as the limitations of science as a vehicle for resolving conflict about chemical regulation. In cases where the available facts do not provide clear answers to regulators' questions, what constructive role can science play? What can be done now to improve the chances that scientists will be able to offer more informative answers in the long run? In answering this question, we carefully evaluate the strengths and weaknesses of the methods used to study chemical carcinogenesis. Also, we find that in some cases the results of scientific studies decrease the controversy about regulatory choices, in other cases they increase it, and in yet other cases they have essentially no impact upon the controversy.

Finally, we evaluate four prominent institutional proposals for reducing or resolving controversy about regulation of potential chemical carcinogens. One such proposal is the scientific consensus conference, where experts are asked to establish a consensus about key scientific questions involved in a policy decision. A second proposal is negotiated rulemaking, in which opposing interest groups negotiate a draft regulation. A third idea is more intensive judicial scrutiny of regulatory decision making to check "unscientific" agency actions and to foster more politically accountable regulatory decisions. The fourth proposal, made in a 1983 report by a committee of the National Research Council, advocated the adoption of uniform risk-assessment guidelines by all federal agencies to help resolve controversy about how to assess the carcinogenicity of chemicals.[8] In Chapter 7 we draw on the case studies described below to analyze the strengths and weaknesses of each of these proposals.

Most actors in the regulatory process are interested in whether chemicals are—from their point of view—regulated too leniently or too strictly. That is not the primary focus of this book. Our interest is in evaluating the process of using science and the advice of scientists in regulatory decision making. We are seeking ways to redefine the science-policy partnership in order to promote public confidence in science and strengthen the democratic character of our regulatory institutions.

• Methods

To better understand the nature of regulatory controversies, we have undertaken in-depth case studies of two specific chemicals, formaldehyde and benzene. For each chemical we present a history of legislative, administrative, and judicial decisions at the federal level, then review the scientific evidence and judgments about the chemical's carcinogenic potential. By linking the discussions of science and policy, we call attention to the political aspects of apparently technical issues and vice versa.

During our three one-day project workshops, scientific, legal, and policy specialists were asked to describe—or, in our jargon, to "map"—the sources of dispute about each chemical. Our first workshop considered how regulators have posed questions to scientists about formaldehyde and benzene. At our second meeting formaldehyde specialists were asked to survey the scientific evidence about cancer risk and illuminate the technical disputes that are of concern to regulators. Our third meeting, attended by benzene specialists, was again devoted to surveying the scientific evidence and conflicts related to regulatory policy. The participants in each meeting were also asked about the prospects for scientific research that would help clarify key uncertainties.

Our case studies, written in draft form prior to the workshops, have been modified substantially in response to discussions at the meetings. (The chairpersons and participants at each of the workshops are presented in the Appendix.) The case studies also reflect data and judgments obtained from numerous personal and telephone interviews.

Throughout the project we tried to avoid making judgments about which scientists were "correct" or which policy options satisfied our personal conceptions of the public interest. The approach was to characterize the regulatory controversies as they emerged in as neutral a fashion as possible. The product of this effort—the case material—comprises the bulk of the book, Chapters 2 through 5. In Chapters 6 and 7 we take a somewhat more normative and evaluative stance about the role of science in regulation, the proper conduct of risk assessment, and the wisdom of the four proposals for institutional reform.

Careful consideration was given to the two chemicals selected for study. Formaldehyde and benzene are important substances; they are useful but potentially toxic chemicals to which all of us are exposed. They provide a rich cross-section of policy controversy since each substance has been the subject of rulemakings at more than one federal regulatory agency. They also provide a rich cross-section of scientific issues, because epidemiological data stimulated the benzene rulemakings and animal bioassay data spurred the formaldehyde rulemakings.

These two chemicals have been particularly controversial. Many other chemical regulations have been issued with less disagreement among scientists, less indecision on the part of regulators, and less involvement on the part of federal judges. Nonetheless, similar questions can be asked for virtually every chemical. How can we best extrapolate responses from rodents to humans? How can we predict responses at very low doses, given responses at very high doses? How can we resolve seemingly conflicting signals from the results of animal and human studies? By listening to how these themes played out for two specific chemicals, we hope to derive some insight into science and regulatory policy for toxic chemicals in general.

There is always a risk, when one relies on a few cases, that the analysis will be distorted by idiosyncratic features. We believe we have successfully avoided these risks for three reasons. First, benzene and formaldehyde were selected in consultation with a steering committee that was knowledgeable about and sensitive to the larger category of cancer disputes. Second, we were seeking cases that represented the widespread confusion about the role of science in resolving regulatory questions. Finally, our examination of a range of similar chemical controversies and the academic literature that has developed about them convinced us that formaldehyde and benzene, considered as a pair, were not aberrations. Indeed, our work has been stimulated and guided by the accounts of other observers.[9]

More fundamentally, the case study method is appropriate for this undertaking, an enterprise that resembles hypothesis generation more than hypothesis testing. We do not claim to have identified phenomena that are universal within some specific class of chemicals or that raise the most important problems in every kind of chemical controversy. Our modest claim is that we have identified in two important cases some interesting hypotheses about the sources of scientific conflict in a regulatory context. We have also suggested some ways society might better cope with such conflicts. For the future we look forward to the "testing" of our hypotheses either through real-world experiments with our ideas or through academic investigation of other chemical controversies. We also are willing to speculate that the sources of scientific conflict revealed in this book are prevalent in a wide variety of technological and scientific disputes that persistently confuse the citizenry.

■ Risk Assessment: Panacea or Obfuscation?

In the case studies that follow, we show how federal regulatory agencies increasingly use risk assessment to bridge the gap between science and public policy. This analytic process is intended to provide regulators and the public with a qualitative and quantitative indication of the toxicity of a chemical or mixture. The methods and findings of risk assessments play a prominent role in the adversarial disputes about toxic chemical regulation.

Cancer risk assessment can be thought of as a four-stage process.

• Hazard identification: a study of the weight of scientific evidence to determine whether or not a chemical or mixture poses a potential risk of cancer to humans.

• Dose-response assessment: a study of the quantitative relationship between the amount of chemical exposure and the incidence of cancer.

• Exposure assessment: a study of the number of people exposed to a chemical and their exposure profiles (concentration, frequency, and duration).

• Risk characterization: a summary of the overall magnitude of risk attributable to chemical exposure, including some reporting of the degree of scientific uncertainty about risk.

Although risk assessment of toxic chemicals is still in its intellectual infancy, an entire consulting industry has arisen to fill the need for risk assessments of toxic chemicals.

In the case studies of formaldehyde and benzene, we describe how risk assessments became so important and how they are used by regulatory agencies to defend policy decisions. The benzene case traces the history of risk assessment to a 1980 decision of the U.S. Supreme Court, while the formaldehyde case illustrates a possible trend toward judicial activism in the review of agency risk assessments. In Chapter 6 we describe the risk assessments performed for formaldehyde and benzene and evaluate these assessments in light of the scientific data, disputes, and uncertainties about each chemical. In Chapter 7 we offer some recommendations designed to improve the honesty, usefulness, and scientific credibility of cancer risk assessment.

2 ▪ SETTING REGULATORY PRIORITIES

IN THIS chapter we investigate how human exposure to formaldehyde became a focus of federal regulation and why the priority-setting decisions of three federal agencies were so controversial and apparently inconsistent. Part of the conflict, which we explore in detail in Chapter 3, seems on the surface to be purely technical, reflecting ambiguities in the scientific data about formaldehyde's adverse health effects. But scientific uncertainty about a chemical's toxicity does not assure heated controversy. There must also be powerful and conflicting interests at stake. Otherwise, no one has any reason to contest either an agency's priorities or its final standards. The fact that formaldehyde was a topic of increasingly intense regulatory debate for almost ten years demonstrates that there were in fact conflicting interests in this case.

On the pro-regulation side was a loose, informal coalition of environmentalists, public health advocates, labor union leaders, and some activist scientists. Their opposition was led by the Formaldehyde Institute, an organization funded by companies with commercial interests in the production and use of the chemical.[1] Although public health and economic concerns surely drove the debate, it would be naive to believe that the "formaldehyde controversy" was solely about formaldehyde. The treatment of this chemical was of special interest because basic issues of precedent were at stake.

The controversy emerged during the period of transition from President Carter to President Reagan. Questions were raised about whether certain "cancer risk assessment guidelines" developed for toxic chemicals during the Carter administration would be implemented by the new political appointees, who had starkly different philosophical attitudes toward regulation. Formaldehyde was a test of whether "generic" guidelines of the sort the Carter administration had offered could be applied credibly to a chemical with a highly complex pattern of scientific data. These guidelines purport to lay out uniform tests for determining what is a carcinogen for regulatory purposes. In particular, because formaldehyde is an animal carcinogen, the guidelines seem to suggest that regulators must treat it as if it was a human carcinogen, despite the absence of positive epidemiological findings. Because this chemical was evaluated by different agencies at different times, we can observe how various legislative mandates, institutional designs, and political forces affected the setting of priorities.

• Sources of Human Exposure

Formaldehyde was first intentionally synthesized in 1868 and has been in commercial production in the United States since 1901.[2] Today it is widely used in industry; more than five billion pounds are produced in the United States annually. More than half is used to make plastics and adhesive resins used in the manufacture of particleboard, fiberboard, and plywood. Formaldehyde also has important applications in textiles (for example, permanent press fabrics), the automotive industry (for example, aluminum casting and rust resisting compounds), the oil industry (as a preservative for oil-drilling muds), and household products (floor coverings, paper towels, and draperies). The direct manufacture of formaldehyde is a $400 million business. According to one estimate, formaldehyde is a component of products that account for 8 percent of the American gross national product (GNP).[3] Given this major economic role, it is no surprise that moves to regulate the chemical have been contested repeatedly.

Everyone is exposed to formaldehyde. The ambient air in rural areas has been found to contain a few parts per billion (ppb), and urban air appears to contain somewhere between 10 and 100 ppb. Formaldehyde in urban air derives primarily from automobile exhausts and other sources of combustion, which emit some formaldehyde directly and also emit hydrocarbons that form formaldehyde in the atmosphere as a result of photooxidation. The air inside buildings seems to contain higher levels of formaldehyde than the air outdoors, in part because formaldehyde gas is released from various building materials, such as particleboard and urea-formaldehyde foam insulation (UFFI). Indoor levels of formaldehyde vary, depending on the nature of the sources and the ventilation rate of the building. Well-insulated homes, homes containing UFFI, and mobile homes have been shown to have airborne levels of formaldehyde ranging from 10 ppb to a few parts per million (ppm).[4]

The highest levels of formaldehyde occur in factories where it is either produced or used and in pathology laboratories, where tissue and bodies are preserved with solutions of formaldehyde (formalin). Levels averaging 1 ppm have been measured in factories that produce formaldehyde, manufacture plywood and particleboard, and make wood furniture. Apparel manufacture has been found to involve average concentrations of 0.5 ppm. Higher levels appear intermittently in laboratory settings.

Formaldehyde as a product of combustion is also present in cigarette smoke.[5] Some scientists regard the formaldehyde in smoke as contributing to the chronic tissue damage sustained by cigarette smokers. Because cigarettes fall outside the purview of the regulatory agencies considered here, this exposure has generally not been at issue in these policy debates.

• Origins of the Controversy

Concerns about human exposure to the chemical are not new. The irritant properties of formaldehyde have long been recognized. Its vapors often cause irritation to the eyes and respiratory tract, and people who are especially sensitive find that their skin begins to itch following contact with cosmetics, paper, or clothing containing even small amounts of formaldehyde.[6] The resulting allergic dermatitis is difficult to define in terms of dose and response because it involves both an initial sensitization and a final elicitation. Although elicitation may not occur below a certain threshold dose, perhaps 30 ppm of formaldehyde in solution, sensitization may occur below this exposure level.[7]

To protect workers from the irritant effects of formaldehyde, the first Occupational Safety and Health Administration (OSHA) standard, adopted in 1972 from the guidelines of the American National Standards Institute, called for maximum permissible doses of 3 ppm as an eight-hour time-weighted average (TWA). This means that during an eight-hour working day continuous occupational exposure is not to exceed an average of 3 parts of formaldehyde per million parts of air. The OSHA standard also set a ceiling dose of 5 ppm, except that excursions up to 10 ppm were allowed for no more than thirty minutes per eight hours.[8]

Many authorities believed the OSHA standard was deficient. For instance, the National Institute of Occupational Safety and Health (NIOSH) recommended to OSHA as early as 1976 that a *ceiling* of 1 ppm should be adopted to assure adequate protection against formaldehyde's irritant effects.[9] As Table 2.1 demonstrates, the United States is one of the more permissive of the world's developed nations in terms of occupational exposure to formaldehyde.

Concern about formaldehyde's irritant effects was heightened when the chemical "move[d] from the workplace to the home, an arena that touches every American consumer."[10] The energy crisis of

Table 2.1 National occupational exposure limits for formaldehyde.

Country	Year	Concentration mg/m^3	ppm	Interpretation	Status
Australia	1978	3	2	Ceiling	Guideline
Belgium	1978	3	2	Ceiling	Regulation
Bulgaria	1971	1	—	Max.	Regulation
Czechoslovakia	1976	2	—	TWA[a]	Regulation
		5	—	Ceiling (10 min.)	Regulation
Finland	1975	3	2	Ceiling	Regulation
Germany, East	1979	2	—	Max. (30 min.)	Regulation
		2	—	TWA	Guideline
Germany, West	1979	1.2	1	TWA	Guideline
Hungary	1974	1	—	TWA	Regulation
Italy	1978	1.2	1	TWA	Guideline
Japan	1978	2.5	2	Ceiling	Regulation
Netherlands	1978	3	—	Ceiling	Regulation
Poland	1976	2	—	Ceiling	Regulation
Romania	1975	4	—	Max.	Regulation
Sweden	1978	3	2	Max. (15 min.)	Guideline
Switzerland	1978	1.2	1	TWA	Regulation
United States	1980	3.7	3	TWA	Regulation
(OSHA)		6.2	5	Ceiling	Regulation
		12.3	10	Ceiling (30 min.)	Regulation
U.S.S.R.	1977	0.5	—	Max.	Regulation
Yugoslavia	1971	1	0.8	Ceiling	Regulation

Source: International Agency for Research of Cancer, *Monographs on the Evaluation of Carcinogenic Risk of Chemicals to Humans,* vol. 29, *Some Industrial Chemicals and Dyestuffs* (Geneva: World Health Organization, 1982), 350.

a. TWA = time-weighted average.

the 1970s caused many homeowners to add insulation and reduce ventilation. From 1975 to 1980, roughly 500,000 houses in the United States were insulated with UFFI.[11] Occupants of some of these houses began to report symptoms such as watery eyes, sore throats, and general discomfort. In October 1976 the U.S. Consumer Product Safety Commission (CPSC) was petitioned by the district attorney of the Consumer Office of Metropolitan Denver to regulate certain home insulation products believed to cause acute health problems among residents. Formaldehyde gas from UFFI was named in the petition. After a staff investigation, CPSC in March 1979 rejected the petition for all insulation products except UFFI. On UFFI, the commission deferred a decision pending the collection of further data.[12]

In October 1979 the Chemical Industry Institute of Toxicology (CIIT), a research organization funded primarily by a consortium of chemical corporations, released the interim results of a laboratory animal bioassay that dramatically escalated the formaldehyde controversy. Interim results revealed that 36 of 206 rats exposed to 15 ppm of formaldehyde had developed nasal carcinomas within eighteen months of exposure. By the end of the thirty-month study, half of the 206 rats exposed to 15 ppm had developed nasal canceer, as had 2 of the 210 rats exposed to 6 ppm of formaldehyde. No nasal cancers were observed in either the control group or the group of rats exposed to 2 ppm of formaldehyde.

The CIIT results had powerful implications for regulatory policy. The risk of cancer from exposure to formaldehyde had not previously been a serious concern. In addition, the Carter administration had recently formulated its generic cancer-policy guidelines for identifying suspected carcinogens. Regulators were instructed to consider any substance that was shown to cause cancer in animal experiments as a cancer risk to humans. This principle received prominence in reports by the Carter administration's Regulatory Council and the Interagency Regulatory Liaison Group (IRLG).[13] Despite this principle, the response of federal agencies to the CIIT results was anything but uniform.

• CPSC and Formaldehyde

Consideration of formaldehyde progressed most quickly at CPSC, where the CIIT results accelerated an investigation already under way. The commission established the Federal Panel on Formalde-

regarding the regulatory responses to different types of evidence of carcinogenicity. But CPSC's cancer policy was overturned in federal court because the agency failed to provide prior notice and opportunity to comment, as required by the Administrative Procedure Act.[25] Rather than enter into protracted litigation, the commission withdrew the proposed cancer rule and, along with the Environmental Protection Agency (EPA), endorsed the cancer policy statement in the previously mentioned report by the Regulatory Council.

From Information to Ban

In June 1980 CPSC became the first federal agency to initiate rulemaking proceedings on formaldehyde after the release of the CIIT results. Although the possibility of cancer risk accelerated the commission's investigation, the rulemaking was originally justified on the basis of irritation. This emphasis is reflected in CPSC's modest regulatory proposal: an information program requiring manufacturers to give specified information to prospective purchasers of UFFI about formaldehyde gas exposure and attendant health effects.[26] The proposal was later withdrawn by the commission, both because of the practical difficulties of such an approach and because of increasing evidence of cancer risk.

The month of November 1980 was quite important in the history of the formaldehyde controversy. The final report of the Federal Panel on Formaldehyde was released, providing further support for pro-regulation forces. After conducting a comprehensive review of data on formaldehyde metabolism, teratology, mutagenicity, carcinogenicity, and epidemiology, the panel concluded that formaldehyde should be "presumed" to pose a risk of cancer to humans.[27] The panel did not, though, make a quantitative estimate of the cancer risk, stating that the data presently available allowed no direct assessment of formaldehyde's carcinogenicity in humans.

The panel's qualitative presumption that formaldehyde is a human carcinogen, offered by a group of scientists, is a classic case of a mixed science-policy judgment. Even though positive animal data are considered by many scientists to be a reliable indicator of human risk, there was a chance that this might be a special case—that is, that formaldehyde might not be a human carcinogen, especially at low doses. The panel's implicit policy judgment was that the risk of societal harm from such a false-positive error was acceptable in light of the risk of public health damage if formaldehyde were treated as not carcinogenic and turned out to be a carcinogen.

Perhaps more important than the panel's report was the defeat of Jimmy Carter by Ronald Reagan in the November presidential election. Entering the presidency on a platform of "regulatory relief," Reagan ordered an immediate freeze on all new federal regulations and established a strict process of centralized regulatory review in the Office of Management and Budget (OMB). It was in this overtly anti-regulation environment that controversy about the alleged cancer risks of formaldehyde was waged. But because CPSC is an independent agency run by five commissioners, each appointed by the president with the approval of the Senate for fixed terms of seven years, its priorities were not immediately affected by the transition from Carter to Reagan. This institutional design insulates the commissioners from White House pressures, as was shown by the formaldehyde case. The commission's rulemaking proceedings are conducted before the entire five-member body and decisions are made by majority vote. When the UFFI case was being considered in early 1981, there were no Reagan appointees on the commission.

The CIIT animal bioassay and the federal panel's report persuaded members of the commission that the cancer risk of formaldehyde exposure might be serious. In December 1980 the Formaldehyde Institute (FI) presented to CPSC epidemiologic studies that found no discernible relationship between formaldehyde exposure and cancer in humans. The FI argued that the positive animal results should be evaluated in the context of these negative results in human studies.

CPSC was clearly not persuaded by the FI's epidemiology. In February 1981 the commission proposed a total ban on UFFI products.[28] Supporting the proposal was a quantitative cancer risk assessment. Based on the CIIT animal data and the "multistage model" of carcinogenesis, CPSC estimated an "upper value of cancer risk" attributable to levels of formaldehyde exposures in homes insulated with UFFI. (As we discuss in Chapter 6, the multistage extrapolation model is among the more popular mathematical models of cancer risk assessment and is the basis of a widely used computer program called GLOBAL 79.)

CPSC's risk estimate was that up to 1.8 additional cases of cancer would occur in humans for every 10,000 residences insulated with UFFI. Expressed differently, the upper-bound estimate was that an individual living in an average UFFI home for nine years after installation would incur an additional risk of 51 in one million of developing cancer from the formaldehyde gas released by the insulation.[29]

The proposed ban on UFFI was based primarily on this risk but also on the apparent irritant effects.

CPSC's cancer risk estimates depended upon several controversial assumptions. In fact, GLOBAL 79's maximum likelihood estimate (MLE) of cancer risk, which is derived from a mathematical "best fit to the data," is "essentially zero" for formaldehyde exposure in UFFI homes. CPSC rejected this estimate in favor of the 95 percent upper confidence limit (UCL) because, it said, the MLE does not account for the possibility that the dose-response curve is linear at low doses. In contrast, the UCL assumes that "the rate of cancer induction will be proportional to the formaldehyde level" at low doses. The commission argued that "prevailing theories of chemical carcinogenicity" offer "a strong argument that at low doses the carcinogenic response is linear with exposure level."[30] (The views of scientists on this issue are analyzed in Chapters 3 and 6.)

CPSC's aggressive rulemaking was striking compared to the virtual silence of OSHA and EPA. Perhaps not accidentally, the Reagan administration was slow to appoint new administrators to EPA and OSHA. The Reagan team was committed to halting new regulations and was in no rush to provide leadership to regulatory agencies.

CPSC's initiative on formaldehyde can be viewed as an attempt by a troubled organization to justify its existence, particularly to potential congressional patrons. At that time the commission was much less politically secure than OSHA and EPA; critics pointed to numerous instances of administrative incompetence and a lack of demonstrable achievements in CPSC's history.[31] Proposals to radically reform or abolish the commission had been frequently proposed and seriously debated in Congress.[32] In this context, the formaldehyde issue was an opportunity for CPSC to achieve a unique regulatory accomplishment in a technical field where it had previously relied on the expertise of other agencies. Strong leadership in cancer prevention might please CPSC's pro-regulation sponsors, even if it would alienate certain segments of the business community.

In April 1981 the Formaldehyde Institute petitioned CPSC to adopt a product safety standard for UFFI instead of a total ban. The argument was that formaldehyde exposures from UFFI could be reduced by requiring training and certification of insulation installers and limiting the use of UFFI to exterior, above-grade walls, with the interiors of the walls painted with an oil-based paint—a technique to reduce the transmission of formaldehyde into interior living spaces. The CPSC ultimately rejected this alternative in favor of a ban, argu-

ing that the proposed standard would not adequately control formaldehyde exposures in homes insulated with UFFI.

Scientific Conflict

During the one-year period between CPSC's proposed ban on UFFI
and its final regulatory decision, a heated debate took place about
the carcinogenic risks of formaldehyde. A report by the Environmental Cancer Information Unit of the Mount Sinai School of Medicine reviewed the interim CIIT results and concluded that
"effective controls should be initiated to reduce or eliminate human
exposure to formaldehyde."[33] That report stimulated the American
Cancer Society to recommend strict regulatory action.[34] In the summer of 1981, Arthur Upton of New York University (NYU), a
former director of the National Cancer Institute, released the results
of additional animal studies. According to Upton, results from the
bioassays at NYU were strikingly consistent with the interim CIIT
findings. In a letter to CPSC, Upton stated that formaldehyde was
"decisively carcinogenic in animals," and "if the carcinogenicity of
formaldehyde is ignored, it would mean that no agent could be
regarded as carcinogenic in the absence of positive evidence in
humans."[35] Upton's letter generated an immediate response from
Joel Bender, chariman of the Medical Committee of the Formaldehyde Institute, who wrote that "to regard formaldehyde as a likely
carcinogen in man is not supportable."[36]

At about this time, a working group of the International Agency
for Research on Cancer (IARC), a respected scientific organization,
analyzed the animal and human data on formaldehyde. The group
found sufficient evidence to conclude that the chemical was an animal carcinogen, but described the epidemiologic studies as inadequate for finding any carcinogenic effects in humans. Indeed,
formaldehyde is like many other chemicals in this respect. Several
hundred chemicals are known to be carcinogenic to laboratory animals, but direct evidence of their human carcinogenicity is either
insufficient or nonexistent. The policy of IARC is to regard such
cases as follows:

In the absence of adequate data on humans, it is reasonable, for practical
purposes, to regard chemicals for which there is sufficient evidence of carcinogenicity in animals as if they presented a carcinogenic risk to humans. The
use of the expressions "for practical purposes" and "as if they presented a

carcinogenic risk" indicates that at the present time a correlation between carcinogenicity in animals and possible human risk cannot be made on a purely scientific basis, but only pragmatically. Such a pragmatical correlation may be useful to regulatory agencies in making decisions related to the primary prevention of cancer.[37]

Some members of the scientific community were disturbed that federal agencies were not moving more quickly to regulate formaldehyde based on the animal results. A letter from Arthur Upton of NYU and I. B. Weinstein of Columbia University to the heads of several federal agencies stressed the necessity of reducing human exposure to formaldehyde, even though confirming epidemiological data were not available.[38] Upton and Weinstein buttressed their position by pointing to the generic cancer-policy guidelines developed during the Carter administration.

Other members of the scientific community argued that CPSC's regulatory analysis gave insufficient attention to epidemiology and made excessive use of the CIIT animal data. John Higginson, former director of IARC, submitted a letter to the commission stating that the epidemiological data on formaldehyde "are insufficient to exclude a minimal risk, but certainly they weigh heavily against the view that formaldehyde constitutes any considerable risk of nasal cancer to man."[39] Responding to CPSC's quantitative risk assessment, Higginson wrote that "exact estimates as to the number of cases of cancer that might be expected to occur in man based on a single rat experiment are silly and simply ignore biological realities."[40]

James Gibson, vice president and director of research at CIIT, also opposed the proposed ban. His letter, submitted just a week before the final vote, argued that the multistage model of cancer risk was only one of four plausible models that could have been used by CPSC analysts. The other three models, noted Gibson, indicated virtually no cancer hazard from UFFI.[41] In particular, he questioned the assumption that the risk of cancer caused by formaldehyde was a linear function of exposure. Because formaldehyde is an "endogenous" chemical (one that is made and used naturally in the human body), Gibson argued that it should not be treated as a foreign substance or poison.

Judicial Resolution

In the midst of all this controversy, the commission voted four to one on February 17, 1982, to ban the use of UFFI in all homes and schools, effective August 10, 1982.[42] Proponents were somewhat surprised that Nancy Stoerts, the Reagan administration's recent choice for chairperson of the commission, voted for the ban.

The commission was immediately sued both by the Formaldehyde Institute and by Ralph Nader's group, Public Citizen, the former opposing the ban and the latter arguing that the ban should have included commercial buildings and other structures. The suits were consolidated in the Fifth Circuit Court of Appeals in New Orleans. Although Nader's group had filed suit in the more liberal District of Columbia Circuit Court of Appeals, the case was assigned to the relatively conservative Fifth Circuit, where the Formaldehyde Institute had filed suit first.[43] Such "court shopping" and "races to the courthouse" have become common phenomena in regulatory litigation.

Regardless of the outcome of the litigation, changing economic circumstances and adverse publicity about UFFI had already taken their toll on the insulation industry. From a peak of 150,000 residential UFFI installations in 1977, the demand plummeted to 3,110 by early 1982.[44] Economic losses were also apparent in the real estate industry, where homes with UFFI had become difficult to sell. Since the cost of removing the foam could easily run to thousands of dollars, owners of UFFI homes found themselves in a painful dilemma.

On April 17, 1983, a unanimous three-judge panel of the Fifth Circuit vacated CPSC's ban of UFFI, citing both procedural error by the agency and a lack of substantial evidence to support its action.[45] The procedural error was the commission's decision to proceed under the informal procedures of the Consumer Product Safety Act instead of the formal procedures of the Federal Hazardous Substances Act (1960). More interesting was that the Fifth Circuit panel was not reluctant to scrutinize the way CPSC had handled the scientific and technical issues.

The judges concluded that the commission's analysis of human exposure to formaldehyde, based largely on data from consumers who complained about UFFI, did not constitute "substantial evidence" for purposes of justifying a ban. According to the court: "The Commission does not explain its reliance on a data base comprised largely of complaint houses. Nor does the agency justify its failure to conduct a study of randomly selected UFFI homes before issuing the product ban."[46]

On the subject of cancer risk, the judges faulted the commission for relying exclusively on the CIIT rat data when other data were available. The opinion stated:

We agree with the agency that the epidemiologic studies cited by the industry do not demonstrate conclusively that formaldehyde poses no cancer risk to man . . . While the Commission correctly notes that the epidemiologic evidence is not conclusive, its exclusive reliance on the Chemical Institute study in its GLOBAL 79 risk assessment is equally unsupportable . . . The Federal Panel's findings that the Chemical Institute study was valid and that formaldehyde should be presumed to pose a cancer risk to man do not authenticate the use of the study's results, and only those results, to predict exactly the cancer risk UFFI poses to man.[47]

Although the UFFI industry was virtually dead, the Fifth Circuit decision became the subject of controversy. A group of health activists at the Massachusetts Institute of Technology's Center for Policy Alternatives criticized the judicial opinion for failing to respect the generic cancer-policy guidelines developed in the Carter administration.[48] Others argued that the Fifth Circuit did not recognize the need for policy judgments in risk assessment when data are lacking.[49] In contrast to these views, the American Industrial Health Council (AIHC)— a business-sponsored organization—hailed the court's decision as support for its charge that the generic cancer guidelines were flawed in several respects. In particular, AIHC highlighted the court's refusal to permit reliance on a single animal study and its criticism of highly imprecise data on exposure.[50] AIHC also drew attention to a footnote in the court's opinion, which questioned CPSC's reliance on the upper confidence limit of risk. One prominent legal scholar, Richard Merrill, dean of the University of Virginia Law School, expressed skepticism about the court's treatment of scientific uncertainty, but nonetheless saw the Fifth Circuit's decision as the beginning of a "new era" in the judicial review of cancer risk assessments.[51]

Key staff members at CPSC were disappointed with the court's review. A majority (three–two) of the commission voted to request a rehearing by the Fifth Circuit, but the Fifth Circuit denied the request.[52] The commission then voted to appeal the decision to the U.S. Supreme Court, but the solicitor general, a Reagan appointee, refused to pursue the commission's appeal in August 1983. Since only the solicitor general can represent the federal government in cases before the Supreme Court, this effectively scuttled the CPSC initiative.

• OSHA and Formaldehyde

The formaldehyde story at OSHA was in many ways the reverse of the CPSC story. The Reagan-appointed leaders at OSHA were determined not to initiate rulemaking on formaldehyde and in fact did not do so until a federal court used the agency's generic cancer rule in part as a basis for compelling such action.

The act of 1970 that created OSHA directed the agency to adopt regulatory standards to assure "safe and healthful" places of employment. Concerning toxic chemicals, Congress provided some minimal guidance to OSHA in Section 6(b)(5): "The Secretary, in promulgating standards dealing with toxic materials or harmful physical agents, shall set the standard which most adequately assures, to the extent feasible, on the basis of the best available evidence, that no employee will suffer material impairment of health or functional capacity."[53]

The ambiguity of the act contributed to extensive litigation, including two cases decided by the U.S. Supreme Court. In the 1980 benzene case a plurality of the Court held that OSHA must show that a chemical poses a "significant risk" of material health impairment before it attempts to regulate exposure.[54] In the 1981 cotton-dust case a majority of the Court held that if a chemical is shown to pose a significant risk, OSHA must reduce exposures to the lowest "feasible" levels, even if cost-benefit analyses might support a weaker or a stricter standard.[55] The impact of these decisions on OSHA's standard-setting practices is discussed in more detail in Chapter 4.

During the Carter administration, OSHA Administrator Eula Bingham promulgated a generic rule for identification and regulation of chemicals suspected of causing cancer.[56] The rule was similar to the IRLG cancer guidelines (which OSHA helped develop) and was designed to accelerate rulemakings on chemicals by giving substantial weight to positive animal studies. Although the rule had been weakened somewhat by amendments and judicial rulings,[57] it was still in effect as a formal agency regulation throughout the formaldehyde controversy.

During the Carter administration OSHA received the interim results of the CIIT study (October 1979) and the federal panel's report (October 1980) on formaldehyde. Despite solid evidence that formaldehyde was an animal carcinogen, OSHA took no action before Bingham left the agency in January 1981. Apparently OSHA and the other IRLG-affiliated agencies (especially EPA) had decided to let CPSC take the lead on formaldehyde.

Auchter's Decision

In March 1981 Thorne Auchter, a construction contractor who had been affiliated with the 1980 Reagan campaign, was appointed administrator of OSHA. From the beginning he made clear that he intended to cultivate a more cooperative relationship with business.

At about the time Auchter took office, OSHA received a report from MIT's Center for Policy Alternatives. The report predicted that between 4 and 5,700 workers would contract cancer each year from formaldehyde exposures permitted by the agency's permissible exposure limit (PEL) of 3 ppm.[58] Even at an exposure level of 0.75 ppm, the MIT report projected 3 to 90 excess cancers per 100,000 workers. Perhaps the key assumption of this report was that the dose-response function relating formaldehyde to cancer risk was linear from a dose of roughly 6 ppm to zero exposure. The authors of the report argued that formaldehyde may have an additive effect with other carcinogenic processes, thus justifying the assumption of a linear dose-response function at low doses.

OSHA commissioned both internal and external reviews of the MIT study.[59] The reviews, which were mixed, criticized the study's reliance on the low-dose linearity hypothesis. (In part the criticism was based on the nonlinearity of the dose-response curve in rats, as we discuss in the next chapter.) Moreover, the statistical model used by the MIT researchers was criticized for producing a poor fit to the CIIT data relative to other models. Auchter ultimately did not act on the basis of the MIT study, although the precise reasons for his inaction were not revealed.

The Infante Affair

The formaldehyde controversy at OSHA became public in the summer of 1981 when an attempt was made to fire epidemiologist Peter F. Infante, then the head of the OSHA office that identifies carcinogens.[60] Infante had angered industry representatives by making statements about the carcinogenicity of formaldehyde. The assistant director of OSHA, Bailus Walker, responded by signing a notice that would have terminated Infante's employment at OSHA. The action was based on Infante's alleged misrepresentation of the agency's position on formaldehyde and his alleged insubordination.

The attempted dismissal sparked instant controversy, including two days of congressional hearings in July 1981 before Democratic Representative Albert Gore's Investigations Subcommittee of the

House Science and Technology Committee. Gore, at the urging of former OSHA head Eula Bingham and other scientists, came to Infante's defense: "If OSHA succeeds in firing Infante, it will be a clear message to all civil servants who are charged with protecting the public health that those who do their job will lose their job."[61] Auchter ultimately rescinded the termination notice and transferred Infante to a less visible position in OSHA.

Labor Seeks Court Relief

The issue heated up again in October 1981 when the United Auto Workers (UAW) petitioned OSHA to adopt an emergency temporary standard (ETS) for formaldehyde. This petition was based on section 6(c)(1) of the Occupational Safety and Health Act of 1970, which states: "The Secretary shall provide . . . for an emergency temporary standard . . . if he determines (A) that employees are exposed to 'grave danger' from exposure to substances or agents determined to be toxic or physically harmful or from new hazards, and (B) that such emergency standard is necessary to protect employees from such danger."[62]

Acting as a loyal supporter of President Reagan's program of regulatory relief, Thorne Auchter in January 1982 rejected the petition. In a letter to the UAW, he argued that the positive cancer findings in the CIIT study occurred at an exposure level (15 ppm) that was well above the prevailing PEL of 3 ppm. In fact, actual exposure levels in workplaces where formaldehyde was used were said to be below 1 ppm in a majority of cases. He also characterized the epidemiological evidence as reassuring because no persuasive evidence of carcinogenic effects had been reported. For these reasons Auchter found that formaldehyde posed no "grave danger" justifying an ETS.[63] The letter did not mention OSHA's generic cancer rule, which supposedly governed Auchter's decision, and in particular, it did not acknowledge that because formaldehyde was an animal carcinogen, the generic rule compelled the agency to treat it as a potential human carcinogen.

About seven months after OSHA's refusal to issue an ETS, the UAW and other activist groups sued OSHA in federal court, arguing that denial of the ETS was an "arbitrary and capricious" use of administrative discretion.[64] The treatment of this lawsuit by the federal district court of the District of Columbia illustrates how a court can influence the rulemaking priorities of a federal agency.

Two and a half years later, in July 1984, the district court remanded the formaldehyde issue to OSHA without compelling any particular form of regulatory action. After reviewing Auchter's reasoning and the accusations of his lack of impartiality, the court decided that OSHA should reconsider the matter. The court was aware that new scientific information had become available between the date of OSHA's denial of an ETS (January 29, 1982) and the date of the court's decision (July 2, 1984). And the White House Office of Science and Technology Policy (OSTP) and EPA had collaborated with the National Center for Toxicological Research (NCTR) to conduct a Consensus Workshop on Formaldehyde in Little Rock, Arkansas. Results from the conference were about to be published when the court's opinion was written.[65]

Although the district court's opinion was written in a highly deferential fashion, it took an important step beyond just remanding the ETS issue to OSHA. The court ordered the agency to formally consider initiating a new permanent rulemaking proceeding on formaldehyde.[66] This subtle form of judicial intervention appears to have been aimed at prodding OSHA into a new rulemaking. In the decision OSHA was ordered to establish a schedule for addressing both the ETS issue and the permanent rulemaking.

Rowland's Decision

By the time OSHA responded to the court's order, Auchter had left the agency for a management position in the private sector and had been succeeded by Robert Rowland, an attorney who had served as chairman of the OSHA review commission and as a manager for the 1980 Reagan campaign in Texas. Like Auchter, Rowland was loyal to the Reagan administration's deregulatory, nonconfrontational philosophy on workers' health issues. Union activists were highly critical of Rowland, both because of his views and because of his sizable investments in the chemical, energy, and pharmaceutical industries. These holdings were legal—Rowland had placed them in a qualified blind trust—but critics claimed he could not make fair decisions on formaldehyde because he owned stock in two companies that made or used formaldehyde.[67] His "recess" appointment (a nomination made while Congress was in recess) was never approved by the Senate, and he held the job for a little more than a year.

In January 1985 Rowland denied the UAW's ETS request and announced a public hearing in which the agency would collect views about whether a new permanent rulemaking on formaldehyde should be initiated.[68] Rowland acknowledged that since formaldehyde was a confirmed animal carcinogen, OSHA was obliged to treat the chemical as a potential human carcinogen. Although cancer was clearly a "grave" health effect, he argued that the magnitude of the potential cancer risk was too uncertain to justify an ETS.[69] Prior OSHA litigation had established that "an emergency standard must be supported by something more than a possibility that a substance may cause cancer in man."[70]

OSHA's Office of Risk Assessment (ORA) had provided Rowland with four estimates of the excess risk of human cancer that might be attributable to formaldehyde exposure. These estimates are summarized in Table 2.2. All were based on the multistage model of carcinogenesis, the same model used by CPSC. While CPSC had placed primary emphasis on the UCL of the model's prediction, OSHA chose to rely primarily on the MLE, the projection that most "closely fit" the actual CIIT data. In a key footnote to the letter, Rowland reaffirmed that OSHA intended to rely on the MLE in making ETS decisions.

The cancer risk estimates in Table 2.2 display a wide variation. At the prevailing 3 ppm standard, the estimates vary by two orders of magnitude. Although even the lowest estimate of risk at 3 ppm is still

Table 2.2 Formaldehyde risk assessments reported in OSHA's ETS ruling: excess lifetime cancers per 100,000 workers.

Exposure assumption	Estimate	OSHA-1	Brown	OSHA-2	Clement
3 ppm	MLE	71	263	5,696	620
	UCL	834	1,819	11,306	930
1 ppm	MLE	0.6	9.1	1,912	23
	UCL	264	606	3,524	130
0.5 ppm	MLE	0.03	1.1	960	2.8
	UCL	132	304	1,959	58

Source: Letter from Robert A. Rowland, OSHA administrator, to Franklin E. Mirer, United Auto Workers, Jan. 7, 1985, mimeo.

Notes: MLE = maximum likelihood estimate; UCL = upper confidence limit (95 percent in each case). All four sets of estimates were based exclusively on the CIIT results and the multistage extrapolation model. OSHA-1 and OSHA-2 used fifth-degree polynomials; Brown used a fourth-degree polynomial; Clement used a third-degree polynomial. All estimates were based on squamous cell tumors except for OSHA-2, which counted both squamous cell tumors (malignant) and polypoid adenomas (benign).

high (71 cases of cancer per 100,000 workers), relatively few workers are actually exposed to 3 ppm on a regular basis. Prior litigation had established that an ETS must be based on actual risks faced by workers, not on hypothetical risks at the prevailing OSHA standard.[71] At the lower exposure levels of 1 and 0.5 ppm, the MLEs vary by several orders of magnitude. Given such huge uncertainty about the effects of formaldehyde, Rowland argued that the extraordinary action of setting an ETS was inappropriate. OSHA stressed that the Consensus Workshop on Formaldehyde had failed to resolve several technical issues that were quite central to assessing the risk of formaldehyde exposure.

Rowland's denial letter drew sharp criticism from the UAW. According to Franklin Mirer, the UAW's director of safety and health, OSHA's rationale could be used to avoid rulemaking activity for any toxic chemical. In particular, Mirer argued that the uncertainties cited by Rowland were inherent in the method of risk assessment and thus should not be used as a rationale for refusing to protect workers from the health risks of formaldehyde exposure.[72]

At OSHA's public hearing on formaldehyde in February 1985, the controversy became even more heated. Suzanne Kessan, an industrial scientist for the International Brotherhood of Teamsters, charged that OSHA had drafted the letter denying the UAW's ETS petition prior to receiving the comments of the National Advisory Committee on Occupational Safety and Health, comments which had been solicited by the agency.[73] According to Michael Silverstein, another UAW official, "while we sit here today and play scientific trivial pursuit, large numbers of workers continue to be exposed to excessive formaldehyde levels."[74] Criticism of OSHA was not confined to labor officials. The toxicology director for Celanese Chemical Corporation, John J. Clary, argued that OSHA's preliminary risk assessment contained numerous defects, including a failure to distinguish administered doses of formaldehyde from effective doses, that is, doses reaching target tissues of laboratory animals. He also argued that OSHA's analysis ignored protective biological mechanisms in humans, such as the mucus layer of the nose, that might be effective at low doses of formaldehyde exposure.

In response to the UAW lawsuit and the federal court order, in April 1985 Rowland initiated a new rulemaking on formaldehyde with an "advance notice."[75] The notice concluded that the existing PEL of 3 ppm was "inadequate," but the justification was based entirely on the chemical's irritant effects rather than on cancer risk.

The notice contained little discussion of the CIIT animal data and only a brief review of the "inadequate" human studies. Rowland indicated that the agency would start drafting a new PEL for formaldehyde. OSHA then petitioned the D.C. Circuit Court of Appeals, which had assumed jurisdiction from the district court, to dismiss the UAW lawsuit. On June 3 the D.C. Circuit denied OSHA's petition and ordered the agency to take "appropriate further action" concerning issuance of a permanent standard by October 1, 1985.[76]

In December 1985 OSHA formally proposed a new permanent standard for formaldehyde. An eight-hour TWA of either 1 or 1.5 ppm was proposed in conjunction with "action levels" of 0.5 and 0.75 ppm, respectively. If exposure levels were found to be at or above the action levels, employers would be required to monitor exposure on a regular basis. The agency also proposed to delete both the existing eight-hour ceiling concentration of 5 ppm and the peak exposure limit of 10 ppm, permitted for up to thirty minutes in an eight-hour day. The proposal was a major commitment of the agency's resources to formaldehyde, even though the agency did not take a decisive position on cancer risk. Instead it requested public comment on whether the tighter standard should be based solely on formaldehyde's irritant effects or also on human cancer risk.

• EPA and Formaldehyde

At EPA two administrators, Ann Gorsuch and William Ruckelshaus, faced the same legislative mandate and roughly the same scientific data, yet reached opposite conclusions about whether formaldehyde should be a rulemaking priority. The simple interpretation is that one of their decisions must have been correct and the other incorrect. A more subtle interpretation is that both decisions were scientifically defensible and that changing political forces and differing policy views generated the disparate outcomes. In fact, we shall argue that managerial incompetence by the Gorsuch team, combined with procedural improprieties in the early formaldehyde deliberations, created strong incentives for Ruckelshaus to reverse the Gorsuch decision. The Ruckelshaus move is particularly interesting because it was accomplished without much immediate tangible cost to the formaldehyde industry and without a retreat from Reagan's program of regulatory relief. Before we examine this hypothesis, it is necessary to review the EPA rulemaking history.

Legislative Mandate

EPA's authority over formaldehyde derived from the Toxic Substances Control Act of 1976 (TSCA). The legislative purpose of the act was "to prevent unreasonable risks of injury to health or the environment associated with the manufacture, processing, distribution in commerce, use, or disposal of chemical substance."[77] TSCA provided EPA with authority to screen new chemicals for safety and to regulate chemicals already in use if they posed an unreasonable risk to health. Section 4(f) of TSCA is an explicit priority-setting provision that directs EPA to give expedited consideration to chemicals meeting certain criteria. The section states:

Upon receipt of (1) any test data required to be submitted under this Act, or (2) any other information available to the Administrator, which indicates to the Administrator that there may be a reasonable basis to conclude that a chemical substance or mixture presents or will present a significant risk of serious or widespread harm to human beings from cancer, gene mutations, or birth defects, the Administrator shall . . . initiate appropriate action under section 5, 6, or 7 to prevent or reduce to a sufficient extent such risk or publish in the Federal Register a finding that such risk is not unreasonable.[78]

EPA has proposed that the seriousness of the harm be judged by the probability that an exposed person will contract the specified health effect. In contrast, the term "widespread" has been taken to refer to the number of persons exposed. Thus, either large risks to individuals or large numbers of exposed persons are, in EPA's view, sufficient to justify designation of formaldehyde as a priority substance under section 4(f) of TSCA.

While TSCA provided some conceptual guidance, important ambiguities remained. The quantitative thresholds for "serious" and "widespread" harm are not specified in TSCA or its legislative history. EPA is apparently expected to exercise policy discretion in establishing these numerical thresholds. More importantly, it is not clear how the agency should reconcile the phrases "may be a reasonable basis to conclude" and the phrase "a significant risk of serious or widespread harm." The former phrase appears to allow less than conclusive evidence of harm while the latter phrase demands something more than just a chance of serious or widespread harm. This problem was particularly severe for formaldehyde because of the scientific conflict over its carcinogenicity.

Gorsuch's Decision

Despite the interim CIIT results of November 1979, EPA moved slowly on a section 4(f) determination during the last year of the Carter administration. In November 1980 the EPA's Office of Toxic Substances (OTS) received the federal panel's report on the carcinogenicity of formaldehyde. In January 1981 OTS determined that formaldehyde might be a candidate for action under section 4(f), and in March of 1981 a *Federal Register* notice was drafted that would support a positive 4(f) determination on formaldehyde.[79]

On May 20, 1981—the day attorney Ann Gorsuch, an appointee of the Reagan administration, took office as EPA administrator—the staff of OTS recommended that she designate formaldehyde a priority substance under section 4(f).[80] Gorsuch responded by directing Deputy Administrator John Hernandez to conduct an independent investigation of the science on formaldehyde before any decision was made. On June 9, Hernandez, a man with considerable technical background, decided that the scientific ambiguities about formaldehyde were substantial and directed the OTS staff to conduct additional studies and collect more data.

During this period representatives of the Formaldehyde Institute and the Chemical Manufacturers Association (CMA) asked to meet with Hernandez to discuss the scientific issues. The groups made it clear that they did not believe that formaldehyde posed the kinds of dangers envisioned by section 4(f) of TSCA. Hernandez agreed to meet, and three meetings were held, on June 19, July 28, and August 14, each attended by several dozen people. Hernandez had directed the acting assistant administrator for pesticides and toxic substances, John Todhunter, to invite appropriate EPA staff and selected outside scientists. The FI was also permitted to invite anyone it thought could contribute to the scientific discussion. Some parties apparently viewed the meetings as "science courts" or "science panels."[81] Hernandez has insisted that the meetings were devoted to scientific issues, not policy recommendations or legal interpretations; no transcripts were made.

The Hernandez meetings were the subject of intense questioning and criticism at congressional hearings the following October. Among others, Democratic Representative Toby Moffett of Connecticut criticized Gorsuch and Hernandez for not inviting scientists from environmental and consumer groups to the sessions. Moffett was also disturbed that some industry lawyers were present at the meetings, creating the further appearance of improper influence over policy.

In September the Natural Resources Defense Council (NRDC) wrote to Gorsuch and requested an explanation for EPA's failure to list formaldehyde as a priority chemical under section 4(f). The letter also contained a threat to sue if EPA did not take prompt action. Gorsuch responded that the agency was nearing completion of its scientific analysis of formaldehyde and would announce a decision by December 5, 1981.

In February 1982 EPA formally decided not to list formaldehyde as a priority chemical under section 4(f). An analysis supporting the decision was contained in a sixteen-page memorandum from Todhunter to Gorsuch. Todhunter acknowledged that formaldehyde might pose some risk of cancer to humans but concluded that the risk was not sufficiently compelling to merit a 4(f) designation. When the memo was released to the public, it became a source of substantial controversy. The team of health activists at MIT's Center for Policy Alternatives criticized EPA's decision on grounds of poor scientific analysis, improper industry influence, and defective legal interpretations. Another commentator described Todhunter's memo as a case study in the "misuse" of scientific data in rulemaking.[82] The House Committee on Science and Technology released a report charging that the memorandum "departed from traditional and widely supported principles for carcinogenic risk assessment."[83] The report also criticized EPA for the lack of peer review of Todhunter's analysis and for the "appearance of impropriety or bias."[84] The formaldehyde case was one example of the kinds of problems that ultimately caused Gorsuch to resign from her position at EPA in the spring of 1983.

Ruckelshaus's Decision

In July 1983 NRDC and the American Public Health Association (APHA) filed suit in the U.S. District Court for the District of Columbia, seeking review of EPA's decision not to consider formaldehyde under section 4(f). These groups and the new leadership of EPA under William Ruckelshaus spent several months attempting to negotiate a settlement of the suit. In November 1983 EPA publicly announced that it would reconsider its 4(f) decision.[85]

In late May 1984, EPA decided to apply section 4(f) to the following two categories of formaldehyde exposure: the manufacture of apparel from fabrics treated with formaldehyde resins and the use in conventional and manufactured (mobile) homes of construction materials containing certain formaldehyde resins. The agency justified the new decision on the basis of quantitative risk estimates.

EPA reported estimates of human exposure to formaldehyde in thirty-three source categories. For each category, the agency estimated the lifetime cancer risk for exposed individuals and the additional cases of cancer that could be expected to occur. The measure of individual risk was used to assess whether the cancer risk was "serious," and the measure of population risk (number of excess cancers) was used to determine whether the risk was "widespread." The mathematical models (multistage and Weibull) used in the exercise produced MLEs and UCLs that generally were within one order of magnitude of each other. Both models fit the CIIT animal data reasonably well, were characterized as compatible with prevailing theories of carcinogenesis, and were described as conservative in the sense that they were not likely to underestimate the actual cancer risks of formaldehyde. EPA, like CPSC, relied primarily on the upper 95 percent confidence limits of the estimates from the multistage model. Although the MLEs of cancer risk were much smaller than the UCLs, EPA said the UCLs were preferred because they presumed linearity in the dose-response function at low doses. That property corresponded with EPA's perception of carcinogenic mechanisms and was favored because it was regarded as conservative.[86]

Table 2.3   EPA estimates of individual lifetime cancer risk for selected sources of formaldehyde exposure.[a]

Source category	No. persons exposed	Multistage model	
		MLE	UCL
Manufacturers, abrasive products	7,000	1×10^{-4}	1×10^{-3}
Manufacturers, asbestos products	3,500	1×10^{-4}	1×10^{-3}
Manufacturers, resins	6,025	3×10^{-4}	2×10^{-3}
Manufacturers, nitrogenous fertilizers	2,250	7×10^{-5}	9×10^{-4}
Funeral service workers	55,000	3×10^{-5}	6×10^{-4}
Manufacturers, textiles	17,800	3×10^{-5}	6×10^{-4}
Manufacturers, hardwood plywood	6,700	3×10^{-5}	6×10^{-4}
Manufacturers, apparel	777,000	2×10^{-5}	6×10^{-4}

Source: Environmental Protection Agency, Federal Register 49 (1984): 21870, 21887–21890.

a. Ranking based on multistage estimate (UCL). Sources with individual risks less than 5×10^{-4} are excluded.

Table 2.3 presents an analysis of formaldehyde source categories according to EPA's estimates of lifetime individual cancer risk. Both MLE and UCL estimates are reported for the multistage model, along with the number of persons exposed. Using these estimates, EPA made the policy judgment that none of the source categories met the "serious" harm test in section 4(f) of TSCA. Apparently EPA decided that the test required an excess lifetime cancer risk of 10^{-2}, or 1 in 100.

Table 2.4 reports formaldehyde source categories according to EPA's estimates of the number of excess cancers. Again the multistage MLEs and UCLs were reported, along with the number of exposed persons. With this information, EPA decided that the top four categories (except for urban ambient air) posed the potential of "widespread" harm envisioned in TSCA. Urban air was excluded because EPA apparently did not trust its own risk estimates (although it recommended that the agency's Office of Air and Radiation accelerate the study of formaldehyde as an air pollutant). EPA did not commit itself to a strict numerical cutoff for widespread harm.

It is impossible to justify the policy reversal from Gorsuch to Ruckelshaus by pointing to changes in the available data. If anything, the case for formaldehyde regulation was slightly weaker in May 1984 than in February 1982 because in the interim several nonpositive epidemiological studies were published.[87]

It is therefore interesting to clarify how the EPA's 4(f) decision

Table 2.4 EPA estimates of excess cancers in the United States from various sources of formaldehyde exposure.

Source category[a]	No. exposed persons	Multistage model	
		MLE	UCL
Residents of conventional (non-UFFI) homes	>100,000,000	20	11,300
Urban ambient air	162,000,000	1	5,346
Residents of new mobile homes	4,200,000	1	588
Manufacturers, apparel	777,000	16	435
Rural ambient air	58,000,000	< 1	140
Residents of conventional (UFFI) homes	1,750,000	1.7	34.7
Manufacturers, wood furniture	59,000	5	34
Wholesale apparel trade	66,400	< 1	22.6

Source: Environmental Protection Agency, *Federal Register,* 49 (1984): 21870, 21887–21890.

a. Source categories that EPA estimates to cause less than 20 excess cancers per year, based on UCL of multistage model, are excluded.

differed from the OSHA and CPSC decisions and to examine why EPA made such an abrupt policy reversal.

Recall that a 4(f) decision under TSCA was not a regulatory decision per se; rather, it was to trigger a decision about whether or not to regulate a substance. In contrast, an ETS at OSHA or a ban of UFFI by CPSC imposed immediate costs on an industry. The question at EPA was simply whether human exposure to formaldehyde created a significant chance of serious or widespread risk of cancer, thereby justifying giving the chemical priority consideration. By the time Ruckelshaus and his appointees decided to reopen the 4(f) issue in November 1983, the politics of EPA regulation had changed. The formaldehyde investigation under Gorsuch had been plagued with procedural improprieties that created embarrassing overtones of pro-industry bias at EPA.[88] The 1984 elections were approaching, and the formaldehyde controversy had become, along with other toxic chemical issues, a symbol of the Reagan administration's alleged insensitivity to environmental concerns. Ruckelshaus was appointed to restore public confidence in the agency.[89] In this atmosphere reconsideration of formaldehyde was a political opportunity. By resolving the 4(f) issue against the wishes of industry, EPA could quiet critics of the administration without taking any immediate and costly regulatory action. At this writing, it is not clear whether or not EPA's policy reversal will result in regulation of formaldehyde exposure. EPA referred the rulemaking question back to OSHA in the case of apparel workers and may do the same to CPSC in the case of UFFI in homes.[90]

• Conclusion

Our survey of agency responses to the CIIT formaldehyde bioassay indicates clearly that a variety of nontechnical considerations played important roles in decisions about setting priorities. How else does one explain the different decisions based on roughly the same data base? Given the importance of nontechnical factors, it is useful to be more explicit about what they were.

At CPSC personal and organizational interests operated in favor of rulemaking. Chairperson Susan King, a Carter appointee and a strong consumer advocate, was looking for ways to expand CPSC's mission into the field of cancer prevention. The CIIT results made formaldehyde a convenient target for King and for other CPSC members and staff who were looking for ways to strengthen the commission's reputation for effectiveness in the eyes of hesitant congressmen and committee staff. Even when Nancy Stoerts was appointed by President Reagan to chair CPSC, the political momentum behind formaldehyde regulation did not wane. Stoerts's vote in favor of a ban on UFFI demonstrated her independence from the White House and may have been an effort to gain credibility among skeptical consumer advocates. Once appointed to the commission, Stoerts could not be dismissed at the pleasure of the president, so she had more flexibility than, say, Auchter at OSHA or Gorsuch at EPA.

During the early Reagan years EPA and OSHA were dominated by the philosophy of regulatory relief, which had been a prominent slogan in Reagan's campaign against Carter. Auchter and Gorsuch perceived their jobs as implementing this philosophy, which meant that to establish any problem as a regulatory priority, even higher *de facto* hurdles had to be overcome. These ideological concerns proved to be far more decisive in the short run than the generic guidelines and rules for priority setting that Carter appointees had developed for suspected chemical carcinogens. Such guidelines involved presumptions that favored regulation on many issues where scientific knowledge about human cancer risk was murky or nonexistent; thus the guidelines were largely ignored by the Reagan regulators.

By ignoring rather than amending or repealing the generic cancer guidelines, the regulators committed a tactical error. The pro-regulation forces turned to lawsuits, and in the case of OSHA, Auchter's failure to consider the generic cancer rule when assessing formaldehyde became grounds for judicial intervention. In fact, the threat and the reality of court-ordered rulemaking became a powerful nontechnical consideration in the priority-setting decisions of Ruckelshaus at EPA and Rowland at OSHA. This judicial interest in priority setting was a relatively new assertion of court power. Federal judges had historically been very reluctant to intrude upon the internal management of priorities at federal agencies.

A related issue is the proper scope for judicial review of cancer risk assessments and priority-setting decisions. Did the Fifth Circuit overstep its technical competence in criticizing CPSC's cancer risk assessment? Were the D.C. District Court and D.C. Circuit Court of Appeals usurping the priority-setting discretion of the Reagan administration on the formaldehyde issue? It is important to consider what federal judges can accomplish when they review agency priority setting. We explore this topic in Chapters 4 and 7.

The formaldehyde controversy also raises fundamental questions about the appropriate role of the White House in regulatory choices. One view holds that federal agencies are responsible only to Congress and that the president should exert relatively little control over their operations. On this view, agencies should codify conservative principles for determining cancer risk and apply these principles consistently in every chemical controversy. A case that departs from such principles is then viewed disapprovingly as the product of political pressure.

An alternative view is that the American people elect the president, who is therefore entitled to shape the priority-setting decisions of federal agencies in accordance with his or her personal philosophy or ideology. From this perspective, strict generic principles for assessment of carcinogens serve only as bureaucratic impediments to the democratic process. The president, it is argued, should have his way unless Congress passes legislation to the contrary or courts find that agencies have behaved in an arbitrary manner.

The case just reviewed raises in a telling way the question of the proper locus of power in regulatory choice. How do we reconcile the responsibility of the executive branch with the policy-setting role of the legislature? To what extent should agencies have some degree of independence from Congress, the courts, and the White House—possibly even becoming a "fourth branch" of government? We return to some of these questions in Chapter 7.

All of these institutional issues aside, the policy history of formaldehyde begins to illustrate important points about the role of science. Formaldehyde was one of the first cases decided under the generic guidelines, and yet the wisdom of those guidelines was strongly challenged in the case. Similarly, in the decisions made by all three agencies, the results of quantitative risk assessments were cited as important rationales.

This history raises some central questions. Were these guidelines and risk estimates based on purely technical considerations? In particular, to what extent did they *reflect*—as opposed to *inform*—policy judgments about how far to err on the side of safety? Just how did the agencies cope with uncertainty when generating risk estimates? Insofar as the estimates were grounded in science, were they based on the best available data and were they consistent with the technical judgments of working scientists? More fundamentally, to what extent were scientists able to directly and honestly answer the questions regulators put to them? Could they tell whether formaldehyde was a human carcinogen and what the precise magnitude of the risk was? What do the answers to these questions imply for our expectations about the ability of science to resolve disputes about carcinogen policy? These are the issues to which we turn in the next chapter, and later in Chapters 6 and 7 as well.

3 ▪ INTERPRETING THE SCIENTIFIC EVIDENCE ON FORMALDEHYDE AND CANCER

FORMALDEHYDE IS a small and simple molecule: one atom of carbon, one of oxygen, and two of hydrogen. Like molecular oxygen, it is a gas at ambient temperatures. But formaldehyde is also a reactive chemical. It can react with and alter other chemicals in air, in liquids, and in the bodies of animals and humans. It can alter proteins and DNA, the basic biochemicals of life. It is conceivable, then, that formaldehyde can affect human health.

During the early and mid-1970s, the chemical was not a rulemaking priority of federal regulatory agencies. There simply was not enough evidence that formaldehyde produced serious adverse health effects at the levels to which most people were normally exposed. As noted in Chapter 2, the situation changed markedly when CIIT's long-term bioassay in rats and mice demonstrated that formaldehyde was a carcinogen in laboratory animals. The generic cancer policy developed during the Carter administration required that positive animal studies be taken as presumptive evidence of a chemical's cancer-causing potential. As we have seen, regulation of formaldehyde did not follow from the CIIT results, in part because of various legal, political, and institutional factors. But disagreement about scientific issues also played a part, including disagreements that went to the heart of the entire attempt to implement a uniform cancer policy. Those scientific issues are the subject of this chapter.

We explore two major issues. First we consider how and why scientists differed in translating the experimental evidence on formaldehyde into estimates of risk to human health. We look at studies at the molecular level, mutagenicity tests, tests of carcinogenicity in rodents, studies of the metabolism of formaldehyde in animals and

This chapter was written with the assistance of Angela Boggs and Scott Wolff.

humans, and the available epidemiological evidence. We find that scientists differ so markedly in their analyses and syntheses of the evidence that they often reach quite divergent conclusions concerning the hazardousness of the substance. We explore some of the reasons for these differences and show how they relate to conflicting opinions about whether and how to regulate formaldehyde.

Second, we examine the complexities of the scientific evidence on formaldehyde to illustrate a fundamental point about chemical regulation. Formal rules that attempt to determine in advance exactly what test results will lead to what regulatory consequences often cannot accommodate the technical judgment and intuition that scientists use to assess cancer risks. This does not mean that generic rules have no role or value, since regulators might deliberately forego some technical sophistication in order to satisfy policy objectives such as predictability and consistency. This chapter, though, reveals the price in foregone scientific judgment that regulators pay when they adhere strictly to generic guidelines.

• The Experimental Biology of Formaldehyde Carcinogenesis

In 1978, CIIT contracted with Battelle Laboratories to perform a long-term bioassay of formaldehyde. The chemical was an ideal candidate for study in many respects; it was produced in great quantity by many manufacturers, many people were exposed to it, and very little was known about its chronic health effects.

Prior to the CIIT bioassay, some preliminary evidence, mostly indirect and mostly published outside of the mainstream American carcinogenesis journals, pointed to the possibility that formaldehyde was carcinogenic.[1] Indeed, in 1978 two researchers acknowledged some early studies but stated that formaldehyde is "generally considered to be noncarcinogenic."[2]

Overall, there has been more agreement than disagreement over the basic methods and results of the CIIT bioassay. Many of the objections that are often raised concerning long-term rodent studies of this type have not been issues in this instance. There is no argument, for example, about the appropriateness of the test animal species or the route of administration of the compound. There is no problem with a high background rate of tumors in the controls and no major problems with diagnosis and enumeration of the induced tumors.[3] At the highest dose level—14.3 ppm—formaldehyde was plainly and unarguably carcinogenic to the rat. This finding was confirmed in experiments by researchers at New York University.[4] But as the data in Table 3.1 illustrate, the results for rats at lower doses and the results for mice are more difficult to interpret.

Dose-Response Relationships

One difficulty in interpreting the results of the bioassay is the large difference in response between the high exposure level and the intermediate level. At 14.3 ppm, 50 percent of the rats developed cancer—specifically, squamous cell carcinomas of the nasal cavity—while at 5.6 ppm only 1 percent did so. That is, when exposure levels differed by 2½-fold, responses differed by 50-fold.

The incidence of tumors at 5.6 ppm was not statistically significantly different from the 0 percent incidence in the unexposed control rats. Yet many scientists, including the authors of the CIIT study, consider the cancers found at 5.6 ppm to be biologically significant. They believe the cancers were in fact the result of formaldehyde exposures, both because they were of precisely the same type (squamous cell tumors) as those appearing at the higher exposure levels and because such tumors are very rare in untreated rats. If spontaneous nasal tumors in rats were not so rare, or if even one such tumor

Table 3.1 *Adjusted* incidence of squamous cell carcinoma of the nasal cavity in rats and mice after inhalation of formaldehyde for twenty-four months.[a]

Formaldehyde concentration (ppm)[b]	Number of tumors/animals at risk[c]	
	Rats (%)	Mice (%)
0	0/208 (0)	0/72 (0)
2	0/210 (0)	0/64 (0)
6	2/210 (1)	0/73 (0)
15	103/206 (50)	2/60 (3.3)

Source: James E. Gibson, ed., *Formaldehyde Toxicity* (Washington, D.C.: Hemisphere Publishing, 1982), p. 297.

a. Six hours/day, five days/week. The study was initiated with 960 Fischer-344 rats and 960 B6C3F1 mice, evenly divided by sex into treatment groups.

b. Target concentrations. Actual average measured concentrations were 0, 2.0, 5.6, and 14.3 ppm.

c. Actual number of animals exposed to formaldehyde up to and including the time when the first squamous cell carcinomas were observed (11–12 months for rats; 23–24 months for mice).

had arisen in one of the 208 unexposed rats in the study, the results at 5.6 ppm would have been quite a bit more controversial.

Two of the *mice* exposed to 14.3 ppm of formaldehyde also developed the same type of tumor. This incidence again was not statistically significantly different from the absence of tumors among the controls, but again the CIIT investigators considered the findings biologically significant: "The spontaneous incidence of nasal tumors in mice is also extremely low . . . Two male mice exposed to 14.3 ppm of formaldehyde in our study developed squamous cell carcinomas in the nasal cavity that were similar to neoplasms observed in rats. This strongly suggests that these tumors in mice resulted from formaldehyde exposures."[5] In contrast, some industry representatives focused initially on the lack of statistical significance in both of these cases. They argued that the results in mice were negative—"there was no statistically significant incidence even at 14.3 ppm"—and in rats were negative for all but the highest dose.[6] This was decidedly the minority view, however; most analysts agreed with the CIIT investigators that the tumors observed in mice at 14.3 ppm and in rats at 5.6 ppm were significant. As we shall see, deciding that formaldehyde is carcinogenic at the *relatively* low exposure level of 5.6 ppm carries important regulatory implications.

A matter of much greater contention—an issue that is absolutely central to the debates about the carcinogenicity of formaldehyde—is what dose-response curve best describes the CIIT data for rats. A closely related question but one that is different in important ways for policy, is how to draw the comparable curve for *humans*. The actual data points from the bioassay of formaldehyde in rats are shown in Fig. 3.1. How should one connect the points shown in the figure? At

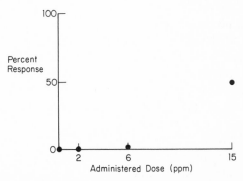

3.1   Dose-response curve from bioassay of formaldehyde in rats.

the extreme, one might consider that the "true" dose-response curve is best approximated by two straight lines: one connecting the points at 14.3 and 5.6 ppm, the other tracing the x-axis to connect the points at 0 and 2 ppm. Extending the first line down to the x-axis posits a threshold for carcinogenic response at about 5 ppm.

A more conventional approach is to assume that dose-response curves for carcinogens have no "threshold dose" (a dose below which no response is expected) and also are linear at low doses. If this is the case, one should be able to plot response as a function of dose and draw a straight line from some observed response down through the origin. Clearly the formaldehyde data deviate from a line within the experimental range, and the question becomes whether to believe the response function is linear at doses below the experimental range.

A second but related question is how to make conservative predictions of low-dose risk, with "conservative" taken to mean "likely to overestimate the risks associated with low doses." Again, a straight line from the response point at high doses through the origin is conservative at low doses if the true function is concave. As an additional measure, the upper 95 percent confidence limit of each observed response is sometimes used to construct a dose-response curve. For example, although the observed response at 2 ppm is 0 percent, this observation stems from only one experiment using about 200 rats. A replicate experiment, or an experiment using a larger group of rats, might reveal a tumor response rate of 1 or 2 percent. Opponents of this conservatism note that one might test 500 or 1,000 rats and *still* find a response rate of 0 percent.

Regardless of whether one uses the observed responses or some upper confidence limit, there remain differences of opinion about how to connect the points. Some scientists believe that the effects of high and low doses of formaldehyde differ qualitatively, not just quantitatively, because they act through different types of toxic and carcinogenic mechanisms. This view suggests a biphasic dose-response curve, with a steeply sloped response in the high-dose region, a portion with a much more shallow—but still nonzero—slope in the low-dose region, and an inflection point somewhere, in this case, between 2 and 5.6 ppm. Such a dose-response function is said to resemble a hockey stick.[7]

Other scientists are inclined to think that the relevant biological and toxicological mechanisms operate at all levels of exposure to formaldehyde and believe that a smooth, continuous, and in this case exponential curve best approximates the true dose-response curve. As described in Chapter 6, there is disagreement among members of this camp as well, concerning the power of the exponential curve and hence the nonlinearity of the relationship. The higher the power, the more convex the curve and the "safer" low doses can appear to be. This issue of nonlinearity therefore has crucial implications for policy. Just how nonlinear is the dose-response curve for formaldehyde? Is it more nonlinear than any other carcinogen? Is it so nonlinear that it suggests the existence of a threshold dose below which no risk of cancer exists? Is it so nonlinear that such a threshold might even be close to 5 ppm? Or can its shape be predicted by analogy with the curves of other "similar" carcinogens?

The dose-response curves for most of the hundreds of other chemicals that have proven to be animal carcinogens are also not known with precision. For practical reasons, chemicals are usually tested at only two or three doses or exposure levels—plus a zero or background exposure level for the control animals. It is not unusual for the lowest dose to result in no detectable excess incidence of tumors. One is therefore often left with a dose-response picture with only one or two nonzero points, through which a wide variety of curves, including one or two straight lines, can be drawn.

To clarify the larger scientific context of this issue, a brief digression is appropriate. For carcinogens that have been tested at a larger number of dose levels, a variety of dose-response curves have appeared. Data from a famous bioassay of vinyl chloride, for example, appeared to fit a "downward curving" concave function, as shown in Fig. 3.2.[8] Another study found evidence of such downward-curving dose-response functions for twenty-three other chemical

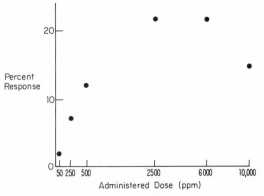

3.2 Dose-response curve from bioassay of vinyl chloride.

carcinogens.[9] The downward curvature means that after a certain point, as the amount of the administered chemical is increased, it becomes relatively less efficient in inducing tumors. For vinyl chloride, the explanation is that the metabolic system that generates the ultimately carcinogenic form becomes saturated. More often such downward curves result from competition between the carcinogenic response and the overall toxic response. Higher doses then become relatively less carcinogenic because they are relatively more toxic, and a dead cell cannot become a cancerous cell. Sometimes downward curvature occurs because a carcinogen appears to be so potent that "it is as though even [the lowest dose] . . . suffices to initiate almost all the cells that are available to be initiated."[10] Whatever the mechanism, these curves have led some analysts to caution that the simple linear extrapolation of carcinogen bioassay data will sometimes *underestimate* the risk at low doses.[11]

On the other hand, data for some other chemical carcinogens appear to fit an upward-curving, convex dose-response function. The data for 2-acetylaminofluorene (AAF) and bladder tumors in mice, for example, produce the curve shown in Fig. 3.3.[12] The results of ethylene thiourea (ETU) and thyroid tumors in rats produce a curve like that shown in Fig. 3.4. The appropriate interpretation of such data is hotly debated. Some take the seemingly straightforward approach: doses that do not induce an excess of cancer in experimental animals are not carcinogenic doses. The "no-observable-effects level" (NOEL) is assumed to be the *actual* no-effects level. For example, researchers at the Food and Drug Administration (FDA) wrote: "ETU was found to be a thyroid carcinogen for the rat at the 250 and 500 ppm dietary levels and a thyroid tumorigen at the 125 ppm level . . . ETU ingestion at the 5 and 25 ppm levels was not biologically deleterious to the

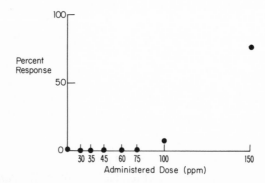

3.3 Dose-response curve for AAF and bladder tumors in mice.

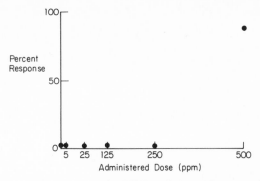

3.4   Dose-response curve for ETU and thyroid tumors in rats.

rat."[13] The investigators believe that above some threshold—presumed to lie between 25 and 125 ppm—the thyroid of the rat is subjected to "excessive pharmacological stimulation," and tumors are not unexpected. But below the threshold dose ETU is not sufficiently toxic to the thyroid, and excess tumors do not appear.

Other analysts use theoretical arguments to reject the notion of a threshold for *any* carcinogen. They argue that if carcinogenesis arises from mutagenesis, and if a mutation can result from a single change in a molecule of DNA caused by a single molecule of a carcinogen, there cannot be a threshold dose below which such an event could not occur.[14] On the other hand, this "one-hit model" cannot be experimentally proven correct, because even the smallest dose of aflatoxin, for example, that is known to cause liver tumors—1 ppb in the diet—contains trillions of molecules of aflatoxin. Certain carcinogens, however, such as radiation, do show linear, nonthreshold behavior over broad ranges of dose.[15] And the compound AAF, shown above to be an unimpressive *bladder* carcinogen at low doses, does not seem to have a threshold for *liver* cancer.[16]

A closer look at the bladder cancer data for AAF raises the question whether the apparent threshold is merely an artifact of the limited time period of the study. As the experimental animals live longer, tumors appear later in life and at lower doses. The dose-response curves shift toward the origin and begin to look as if they do not have a threshold; as Fig. 3.5 shows. This is a commonly observed phenomenon. Low doses often reveal their carcinogenic effects only after a long time.[17] This is one reason that carcinogen bioassays now routinely cover the animals' natural life spans. Earlier studies often ended at eighteen months and thus failed to reveal these senescent tumors.

Some analysts maintain that this "time-to-tumor" effect should

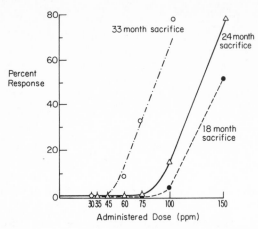

3.5 Dose-response curves for different time periods for AAF and bladder tumors in mice.

form the basis for a "working threshold."[18] They argue that there is no risk from doses so low as to induce excess tumors only after four years of exposure, for example, if an animal's natural life span is only three years. Critics counter that positing such a working threshold is no easier than attempting to predict an absolute one. Extrapolations must still extend into regions without data, using a mathematical model that is more or less speculative.

The data on AAF and bladder cancer also show that extremely nonlinear dose-response curves for carcinogens are known, for example:

Dose of AAF in diet	Incidence of bladder tumors in mice
75 ppm	1 percent
100 ppm	16 percent
150 ppm	77 percent

This dose-response curve is extremely nonlinear, like that of formaldehyde! Interestingly, the nonlinearity of the curve for AAF was remarked upon by the investigators, but no issue was made of it.[19] Presumably this is because AAF is not an item of commerce, people are not exposed to it outside of the laboratory, and therefore no regulatory questions are hanging in the balance.

What this review suggests is that the existing state of theoretical and empirical work on chemical carcinogenesis is unlikely to provide a clear and compelling answer to the question whether there is a threshold in the dose-response function for formaldehyde. The experimental data are various and subject to divergent interpretations. None of the arguments is strictly scientific. Scientists debating the question whether there "is" a threshold for formaldehyde in rodents are actually addressing the mixed science-policy question whether, given the evidence and the consequences of various mistakes, formaldehyde ought to be treated for regulatory purposes *as if* it exhibited such a threshold in humans.

Different Mechanistic Interpretations

Given the limited data, scientists have had to resort to various mechanistic hypotheses to justify their predictions of the shape of the formaldehyde dose-response curve near the origin. Some argue, for example, that the dose of formaldehyde administered is not the same as the dose delivered to the target tissue, and that this has important implications for low-dose extrapolation of risk. Others assume or attempt to demonstrate that the mucus produced by the nasal epithelium (lining) protects against low levels of formaldehyde. Some analysts argue that high doses of formaldehyde are both toxic and carcinogenic, but that low doses, which are not overtly toxic, would not be expected to be carcinogenic. Others counter that benign tumors were observed in rats even at the lowest level of exposure to formaldehyde—suggesting that adverse effects occur even at low levels. There is also the question of whether "endogenous formaldehyde" has any relevance to the safety of low doses of formaldehyde. We will consider all of these issues and then turn to two others— definition of dose and site specificity—that relate to the epidemiological evidence.

Those who believe that formaldehyde's dose-response curve is likely to be nonlinear at low doses argue that the high cancer incidence at 14.3 ppm is attributable to the acutely and chronically irritating effects of formaldehyde at this level. This dose clearly irritates the nasal lining, destroying the normal mucociliary clearance process, denuding the epithelium, and generally causing much more damage, and different kinds of damage, than would occur at lower doses, with the normal barriers and defense mechanisms intact. This leads some scientists to accept the notion of a no-effect threshold at more or less the nonirritation level.

The opposite camp responds that although the incidence of tumors in laboratory animals was nonlinear with dose, there is no good reason to dismiss the carcinogenic potential of formaldehyde at exposure levels experienced by humans. This side notes that the lowest level producing carcinomas in rats—5.6 ppm—is only twice the current occupational exposure limit for a time-weighted average; that there is some evidence of chronic irritation in rats exposed to 2 ppm; and that the evidence that 2 ppm does not cause cancer in rats derives from only one experiment with only 200 rats.

The general disagreement, then, is over whether some of the important underlying processes leading to tumors operate differently at high doses than at low doses. Indeed it is difficult to look at the experimental data prima facie and argue against this general notion. *Something* in the carcinogenic responses of animals exposed to 5.6 ppm must differ from those of animals exposed to 14.3 ppm. If not, one would expect to see either a lot more tumors at 5.6 pm or a lot fewer at 14.3 ppm. The debates center on just what the differences are, and whether and how they should be factored into predictions of tumor yields at the lower exposure levels experienced by humans.

Delivered doses. Some scientists, notably the principal investigators of the CIIT bioassay,[20] argue that gross irritation from high doses of formaldehyde causes both biological and physical changes in the epithelium of the nasal cavities of the rat, so that a larger proportion of the compound is able to penetrate and thus damage the basal cells. The actual "delivered dose" of formaldehyde, they hypothesize, is disproportionately larger at high exposure levels than at lower, less irritating levels.

Early evidence published by CIIT scientists, however, seemed to be inconsistent with this hypothesis. One group of researchers measured the radioactive carbon—^{14}C—incorporated into the nasal mucosa of rats inhaling various levels of formaldehyde. Formaldehyde labeled with ^{14}C was absorbed at rates *directly* proportional to the exposure level, from a concentration of 15 ppm to as low as 0.6 ppm. In other words, the ratio of administered dose to delivered dose was identical for all levels of formaldehyde examined. The investigators also noted: "It is important as well that the amount . . . absorbed did not appear to vary following pre-exposure [to formaldehyde] . . . Hence, these findings, which are based on single exposures, may also be relevant to the chronic toxicity of formaldehyde."[21]

In another series of experiments, researchers examined an indirect indicator of DNA alterations in the nasal mucosal cells of rats exposed to formaldehyde. They determined that the yield of these formaldehyde-induced changes—DNA-protein cross-links—increased linearly with airborne formaldehyde concentrations of 0, 2, 6, 15, and 30 ppm, although the increase from 0 to 2 ppm was not statistically significant.[22]

More recent findings, however, tend to support the hypothesis that the delivered dose of formaldehyde can be nonlinear relative to the administered dose. When rats were exposed to various levels of ^{14}C-labeled formaldehyde, although the amount of ^{14}C incorporated into *protein* of the nasal mucosa was a linear function of exposure, the amount incorporated into DNA showed a discontinuity at 2 ppm of formaldehyde. At this exposure level the delivered dose was about four times lower than would have been expected from a straight-line extrapolation from the higher exposures.[23]

Although these data lend credence to the view that the delivered doses at low exposures are lower than expected, the data do not show nonlinearities in the range of 6 to 15 ppm—the range in which tumor rates were observed to be strongly disproportional to exposure levels. Furthermore, although a case can be made that the dose delivered to DNA may be a valid predictor of genotoxic responses such as mutations, there is much less evidence upon which to argue that such a measure would predict the entire range of toxic responses to formaldehyde, such as irritation, adverse effects at the cell membrane, and cell death.

We discuss the delivered-dose hypothesis in more detail in Chapter 6; some scientists are inclined to use this data in quantitative risk assessment while others consider such use premature.

Mucus. One group has argued that mucus might be expected to protect epithelial cells from exposure to low levels of formaldehyde: "In the rat nasal passages the mucus is continuous over most of the respiratory epithelium. Thus . . . if the rate of binding and removal of formaldehyde by the mucous layer were equal to the rate of delivery of the gas to the exposed surface, then one could reasonably assume that the underlying epithelium would not be exposed . . . Assessment of the effectiveness of the mucus or other potentially protective 'barriers' may permit estimation of a threshold or no-effect level."[24] The group's published studies, however, only investigated a level of 15 ppm of formaldehyde, at which there was clear impairment of mucociliary function in the noses of rats. In a relatively old study, formaldehyde levels as low as 0.5 ppm were found to (reversibly) halt ciliary movement and the attendant transport of mucus in the tracheas of rats.[25] Later work has shown that absorption, metabolism, and excretion of formaldehyde are in fact directly proportional to the exposure level.[26]

The notion that mucus is protective against low levels of formaldehyde has been challenged on other grounds as well. One investigation noted that the nasal mucus layer is more properly thought of as a number of streams rather than a blanket, and that these streams are not completely overlapping and are not impenetrable.[27] Others, referring to extrapolations to humans, argue further that even if an intact mucus "barrier" afforded some or even complete protection against low levels of formaldehyde, such a barrier would be unlikely to be intact in cigarette smokers, people exposed to other irritants, people with colds, and other sensitive groups.

Hyperplasia. Increased cell turnover (death of existing cells and creation of new cells), or hyperplasia, has been proposed as another explanation for the disproportionately high number of tumors at high doses of formaldehyde. This is a more traditional and more widely accepted explanation than the concepts of delivered dose and mucus barrier noted above. As one group of researchers noted, "The fact that only exposure concentrations associated with squamous cell carcinoma in rats and mice resulted in increased cell proliferation lends strong support to the hypothesis that increased cell proliferation is a critical event in formaldehyde carcinogenesis."[28] The European Chemical Industry Ecology and Toxicology Centre (ECIETC) stated: "There are strong indications that nasal cancers develop only at concentrations that produce chronic tissue irritation. The rapid cell proliferation induced by a cytotoxic and irritating dose may facilitate the occurrence of mutagenic effects and may overcome the effectiveness of DNA-repair."[29]

Two notions are being expressed here. First, increased cell proliferation, because it involves *more* replication of DNA, would lead to greater opportunities for mutagenesis and other DNA damage. Second, faster replication of DNA may outpace the normal attempts of DNA-repair enzymes to correct the damage.

Critics point out, though, that the protective role of DNA repair in human carcinogenesis is not yet firmly established.[30] Even the more general concept that increased cell proliferation is required for carcinogenesis is, they argue, less than well established. There is support for this requirement in experimental systems *in vitro*, but the *in vivo* evidence is so far limited to carcinogenesis of the liver. By this reasoning, carcinogenesis in normally *nonproliferating* organs, such as the liver or brain, might well be strongly dependent upon the qualitative change afforded by induced cell proliferation. But carcinogenesis in normally proliferating tissues, including the nasal epithelium, is, in this view, unlikely to be crucially dependent only upon quantitative changes in proliferative rates.

Thus some critics concede that there is a dose-dependent increase of cell proliferation in the nasal epithelium of animals exposed to formaldehyde, and even that this cytotoxic response has a threshold dose below which no such increase would be expected, but they allow only that this may make low doses of formaldehyde relatively less carcinogenic, certainly not noncarcinogenic. According to this view, there is no threshold for carcinogenesis itself on the basis of cell proliferation, since the cells of the target tissue normally continue to proliferate. The DNA of these normally proliferating cells would still be reactive to, and potentially damaged by, formaldehyde.

Some researchers have argued that the experimental evidence can be read as consistent with this position. The effects of formaldehyde that operate through cell proliferation may make the dose-response curve nonlinear at high, cytotoxic doses, while the genotoxic effects on DNA imply a linear relationship at lower, noncytotoxic doses.[31] Alternatively, these effects might produce a discontinuous dose-response curve, with one steeply sloped linear segment at cytotoxic doses, and another linear segment of shallow slope at noncytotoxic doses.

Some data on increased cell proliferation in response to increased levels of formaldehyde appear to account for at least some of the nonlinearity in the dose-response curve.[32] Can it account for all of it? This is difficult to determine. It is not easy to quantify increases in proliferation, and the results are highly dependent upon the precise conditions of the assay. Under a variety of assay conditions, the researchers repeatedly found large increases in cell proliferation in rats following exposures to 6 or 15 ppm of formaldehyde relative to exposures to 2 ppm and below. Similarly, cell proliferation in mice increased after exposures to 15 ppm, while exposures to 6 ppm and below showed no effect. But in one set of experiments, rats exposed to 15 ppm actually showed *lower* rates of cell proliferation than did those exposed to 6 ppm, while in another set of experiments, rats exposed to 12 ppm for three hours a day showed proliferation rates three times greater than those observed in rats exposed to 6 ppm for six hours a day. In the latter series of experiments, a two- to three-fold increase in cell proliferation relative to controls was noted in rats exposed to as little as 3 ppm for twelve hours per day.

The prevalent view is that it is not yet possible to quantify increases in cell proliferation as a function of formaldehyde exposure levels. It is also widely held that although increased cell proliferation will result in a higher rate of tumor formation, it will not in and of itself *cause* tumor formation. A minority view, as ascribed above to ECIETC, is that formaldehyde-induced tumors arise *only* following formaldehyde-induced increases in cell proliferation.

Squamous cell metaplasia. Still another argument advanced in support of a qualitative difference between high and low doses of formaldehyde is based upon the *pathological* changes caused by the higher doses. The reasoning is that increased cell proliferation—hyperplasia—is only the first step in a series of drastic changes that any irritant produces in the normal cellular architecture of the nasal epithelium. Further change is that the normal ciliated epithelial cells are replaced with abnormal, nonciliated squamous cells. This process, termed squamous cell metaplasia, is a classical adaptive response of epithelial cells to chronic insult. In cigarette smokers, for example, the bronchial epithelium is replaced by squamous cells. This condition is often considered to be precarcinogenic in the sense that if carcinomas subsequently arise, they do so within the metaplastic areas.

For formaldehyde-induced carcinogenesis, then, the argument is as follows:

- The only tumors experimentally attributable to formaldehyde gas are squamous cell carcinomas

- Squamous cell carcinomas can arise only from squamous cells

- Squamous cells arise in the nasal cavity epithelium only as a response to chronic irritation

- Therefore there is a threshold for an irritant-carcinogen such as formaldehyde, which is the observable and theoretically predictable threshold for irritation.

The ECIETC employs this reasoning: "When carcinogenic response is limited to the induction of squamous cell carcinomas in the nasal passages, there is a distinct possibility that squamous metaplasia is essential for their subsequent development. Where exposure is so low that metaplasia does not occur it is unlikely that tumors will develop."[33] The ECIETC argues that formaldehyde is not like some other chemicals, such as some alkylating agents, that are known to induce other types of nasal cancer such as adenocarcinomas. These other chemicals do not appear to induce metaplasia as a prelude to tumor development and are more properly regarded as carcinogenic at even very low doses.

Some analysts agree with this line of reasoning but wonder how low formaldehyde exposures must be to not cause metaplasia. Certainly metaplasia was most frequent and severe in the CIIT rats exposed to 14.3 ppm, but some degree of metaplasia was evident even at 2 ppm.[34] Furthermore, some researchers found that *monkeys* as well as rats developed squamous cell metaplasia in the nasal epithelium when exposed to 3 ppm of formaldehyde.[35] The animals showed no signs of metaplasia at 1 ppm.

For purposes of regulatory policy, this argument has been used to suggest that ambient exposure levels well below 1 ppm—such as would fall within EPA's purview—are likely to fall below the threshold for chronic irritation and metaplasia, and therefore below the thresholds for all significant health effects (except possibly for allergic responses). But for occupational exposures, especially those near the allowable TWA limits of 3 ppm and ceilings of 5 ppm and 10 ppm, the experimental evidence suggests that some degree of metaplasia, and its more serious sequelae, may result.

Has chronic irritation in general been shown to be important in carcinogenesis? The answer for some experimental systems is a qualified "yes." If one applies a solvent such as turpentine to the skin of mice, in the absence of any other treatment, one observes irritation but no tumors. But if the skin has been first exposed to an "initiating" (genotoxic) chemical, the subsequent application of the irritant turpentine does result in tumors—many more tumors than would result from exposure to the genotoxic chemical without the turpentine. In this case, turpentine is regarded as a cancer promoter.

There is some indication that lung cancer rates can also be enhanced by promoter substances. Exposure to irritating dust or to urethane appears to promote lung cancer initiated by radiation.[36] Combinations of some chemicals appear to act synergistically in causing respiratory tract tumors in experimental animals[37] and in humans.[38] And formaldehyde, although apparently not carcinogenic per se in hamsters exposed to 10 ppm, does appear to increase the yield of lung adenomas in hamsters induced with the potent carcinogen diethylnitrosamine. The author of this study concludes: "Formaldehyde may act as a cofactor in chemical carcinogenesis in the respiratory tract."[39]

As part of this controversy, some refer to an experiment performed at NYU.[40] The investigators explored the possibility that a low level of hydrochloric acid (HCl) might react with formaldehyde to form the known nasal carcinogen bischloromethyl ether (BCME). The experimenters exposed rats to either 14 ppm of formaldehyde or 10 ppm of HCl or a combination of the two gases at these concentrations. All exposures were for six hours per day, five days per week, for the lifetime of the animals. The rats exposed to HCl plus formaldehyde did not appear to be at greater risk for nasal cancer than rats exposed to formaldehyde alone. Apparently the potent nasal carcinogen BCME did not form under these conditions, and the irritant but nongenotoxic HCl did not enhance the tumorigenicity of formaldehyde.

Some critics of this study have faulted it for testing HCl only at a concentration that is well below the dose generally considered to be irritating. The authors point out, though, that the study was not intended to explore the irritation hypothesis, and they agree with their critics that it does not disprove that notion. No investigators have gone on to test HCl at high concentrations, so direct support for the hypothesis is lacking.

To date, then, it is not known whether formaldehyde is "just" an irritant or an irritant and a carcinogen. Some consider the latter to be more likely, because formaldehyde is an established mutagen (as discussed below) that alters DNA in ways suggesting it can *initiate* carcinogenic actions even in the absence of any irritant, promoting effects.

Benign tumors. We have focused so far on the malignant tumors—squamous cell carcinomas—that developed in rats exposed to formaldehyde in the CIIT experiment. But some benign tumors—polypoid adenomas of the nasal cavity—were also observed in the study. The dose-response function for these tumors, as shown in Table 3.2, is difficult to interpret, primarily because fewer tumors were observed at the higher dose. The number of these tumors in each of the exposed groups is not statistically significantly different from the single tumor among the controls, but there is a significant ($p < 0.05$) trend in the rate of tumors for male rats. Are these particular responses of biological significance?

The CIIT investigators consider this data to suggest that polypoid adenomas "represent a formaldehyde-enhanced lesion."[41] Some analysts take these results very seriously, pointing to these tumors and the two malignant counterparts (adenocarcinomas) found at 14.3 ppm as evidence that formaldehyde is carcinogenic in rats at exposure levels as low as 2 ppm.[42]

Table 3.2 Incidence of polypoid adenomas in the CIIT experiment.

Sex	Formaldehyde concentration (ppm)			
	0	2.0	5.6	14.3
Male	1/118	4/118[a]	6/119[b]	4/117
Female	0/114	4/118	0/116	1/115
Combined	1/232	8/236	6/235	5/232

Source: Adapted from J. A. Swenberg and C. J. Boreiko, "Appropriateness of Polypoid Adenoma for Quantitative Risk Assessment" (Research Triangle Park, N.C.: CIIT, Mar. 7, 1985), mimeo.

a. Two tumors in this group were judged by pathologists to be borderline hyperplasia.

b. One tumor in this group was judged by pathologists to be borderline hyperplasia.

Others, however, consider 2 ppm of formaldehyde a noncarcinogenic dose for rats. This is the case, strictly speaking, in that "carcinogenic" means able to induce malignant tumors, and none were observed at 2 ppm.[43] The overall issue, though, is how much importance to attach to benign tumors that are apparently formaldehyde enhanced.

Some argue that benign tumors are serious in and of themselves, whether or not some fraction of them progress to malignancy. According to this view, benign tumors are benign only in the sense that they do not metastasize; some can grow large enough to obstruct organs or airways and can even be fatal. In the CIIT study, some of the polypoid adenomas had grown into and obstructed the nasal cavity. In 1984 EPA took the following view: "These benign tumors did not exhibit a dose-response relationship. However, because this type of benign nasal tumor is rare it is likely related to formaldehyde exposure. EPA considers the benign tumors observed in the CIIT rat study to be an indication of significant pathology at low doses."[44]

The usual focus of debate about benign tumors is whether they progress to malignancy. The CIIT investigators state that "there was no evidence of progress from polypoid adenoma to squamous cell carcinoma."[45] There is little reason to suspect this particular progression on the basis of pathology of the two types of tumors, however, and there is no serious debate on this point. As noted above, some analysts regard the two adenocarcinomas in the CIIT study as evidence that the adenomas progress to malignancy.[46] In contrast, the Formaldehyde Institute claims there is "no evidence of progression to malignancy" and states that the role of the adenomas "in the carcinogenic progress is unclear, but in any event, they do not reflect as severe an effect as the malignant tumors."[47] We revisit this controversy in Chapter 6, where we examine the role of benign tumors in quantitative risk assessment.

Endogenous formaldehyde. A final mechanistic argument about formaldehyde is that "natural is safe." Many scientists believe that formaldehyde is a natural, normal, and essential metabolite—a product of normal chemical processes in all animals, including humans. Some take this to mean that there must be a nonzero level at which *exogenous* formaldehyde carries no risk. For example, in the opinion of the National Research Council's Committee on Aldehydes, "formaldehyde is a normal metabolite and a vital ingredient in the synthesis of essential biochemical substances in man and thus in small quantities is not toxic."[48] Further, it is argued that because enzyme systems in the body exist to transfer formaldehyde from reactions that produce it to reactions that require it, the same systems would take up exogenous formaldehyde, thus limiting its ability to directly react with and damage DNA. One group of investigators states: "In the case of this animal carcinogen, there is some normal metabolic mechanism for handling it in all plant and animal species. This suggests the reality of a no-effect level."[49] For the general case, another researcher has argued:

There are two instances of biological circumstances which unequivocally dramatize the concept of a threshold level of carcinogenic effect . . . Estrogens and androgens are carcinogenic for experimental species, and in the case of estrogens, the occurrence of disease in humans has been documented. In the case of the synthetic estrogen stilbestrol and the naturally occurring estrone, cancer has been observed only after the administration of large doses of these agents. Estrogenic hormones are ever-present at subthreshold levels in the earth's population. The second instance relates to the universal occurrence of certain trace metals, such as nickel and chromium, in the bodies of man. In both animals and man these elements have been shown to be carcinogenic at high dose levels. Their physiologic presence, however, is unaccompanied by any demonstratable abnormalities.[50]

Interestingly, the other side uses the example of estrogens to make the opposite point: "Estrogen is an acknowledged bionutrient and endogenous substance, and yet, an established carcinogen. In addition, animal data and human epidemiological data both showed reduced frequencies of breast tumors in ovariectomized females, indicating that estrogens, even while performing their necessary biological functions at physiological levels, simultaneously contribute to the 'background' incidence of breast cancer. The risks appear to rise continuously with dose and without any evidence of threshold."[51] According to this view, endogenous formaldehyde might contribute to the "background" cancer rate in the population. One researcher makes the point more generally: "Chemicals are not known to induce any tumors that do not naturally occur. Therefore, some of the background incidence of tumors, cancers in the population may well be due to these critical, important, necessary trace elements, hormones, and so forth."[52]

It is also possible that this entire controversy is misdirected. Laura Green and Angela Boggs have argued elsewhere that there is really no such thing as endogenous formaldehyde.[53] Instead, what appears to be formaldehyde is actually only one carbon unit bound into larger structures that react (hydrolyze) upon laboratory analysis to generate formaldehyde molecules *in vitro*. In other words, there is no *free* endogenous formaldehyde. Exogenous, free formaldehyde is in chemical equilibrium with these bound units, but the two are quite unlikely to be equivalent toxicologically.

The issue of endogenous formaldehyde illustrates the mixture of values and evidence in the general controversy over formaldehyde. Antiregulatory analysts argue that low levels of formaldehyde must be "safe" because they are natural; pro-regulatory analysts counter that this is a non sequitur. Meanwhile, the underlying *science* on endogenous and exogenous formaldehyde plays a relatively small role in the positions of the protagonists.

On the Use of Mechanistic Information

Recently described mechanisms, insofar as they are biologically accurate, suggest that low doses of formaldehyde are less risky than standard risk assessment methods predict. The presence of mucus in the nasal cavity is said to be protective against low doses. The delivered dose of formaldehyde to target tissues is said to be less than proportionate to the administered dose at low levels. Hyperplasia and metaplasia have been said to be necessary precursors to neoplasia, suggesting that at low doses none of the former, and therefore none of the latter, will occur. As we shall see, some parallel mechanistic considerations accompany scientific disputes about benzene, with the same effect of causing low doses to appear relatively less risky than might otherwise be predicted.

As a logical matter, the use of mechanistic information does not have to lead to risk estimates that are lower than the predictions by standard methods. Mechanistic considerations can be advanced that imply enhancement of risk. For example, humans might be much more sensitive than rats to low doses of an airborne carcinogen, perhaps because of differences between the species in the structure and function of the nasal epithelia. Moreover, our later discussion of peak exposures to formaldehyde suggests that cumulative dose—the standard measure of dose—may not always have a conservative effect on risk estimates. But insofar as standard methods are designed to be extremely conservative, mechanistic considerations often lead to lower risk estimates.

The debate about incorporating mechanistic information into risk assessment and decision making illustrates the mingling of scientific and political reasoning. Some environmentalists argue, for example, that mechanistic research is often done in industrial laboratories or is supported by corporations. They see the emergence of mechanistic research as a strategy by industry to reduce or eliminate regulatory requirements. Industry, with its large fiscal and technical resources, they argue, is able to dominate the debates. Public health advocates argue that because so little is understood about the biological mechanisms of chemical carcinogenesis, case-by-case incorporation of mechanistic information produced by industrial scientists may lead to inappropriate relaxation of regulatory requirements. Even for those cases in which enough might be known to allow the use of some metabolic or mechanistic data, the use of such data could create dangerous precedents.

On the other hand, some scientists—including many representatives of industry—view research about cancer mechanisms as a way to put risk assessment and regulation on a sounder scientific footing. They are frustrated by the opposition to use of such information.

A third view is that mechanistic research is too often a reaction to regulatory pressures. For this reason views about the utility of such research are prematurely polarized which detracts from the long-run effort to better understand the relationship between chemical exposures and human cancer. This view holds that basic research into carcinogenic mechanisms—a program supported by industry, government, and environmentalists—is required to generate knowledge about the biology of carcinogenesis.

The points are well illustrated in a heated exchange of letters to the editor of the journal published by the Society of Toxicology.[54] The letters were occasioned by an article on the positive results of "delivered dose" investigations. As discussed above, the investigators, all from CIIT, had found that one measure of formaldehyde's effects upon DNA—DNA-protein cross-links—increased less than proportionally with increasing dose, and they stated that such mechanistic information was important for the assessment of carcinogenic risk. Their critics were from CPSC, EPA, and the National Center for Toxicological Research.

The letters showed disagreements on a range of issues, from strictly technical points to views about how society should make regulatory decisions. The critics of the article began by questioning how the CIIT researchers could say what the *implications* of DNA-protein cross-links were for risk assessment. They argued that "the mechanism of formaldehyde carcinogenesis is presently unknown," that "formaldehyde may contribute to carcinogenesis in more ways than directly damaging the genome [DNA]," and that "'the relationship between DNA-protein cross-links and carcinogenesis has not been defined for formaldehyde or other chemical carcinogens."[55] The researchers responded indirectly, stating that "uncertainties in risk extrapolation mandate rather than preclude the use of all available biological data." They argued further that "it seems to us that the burden of proof falls on those who would disregard mechanistic information, rather than on those who would utilize it together with other data to assess risk."[56]

The rift between the two camps is deep. The letter from the critics concluded: "Although . . . [the CIIT] paper is an interesting first step in defining a molecular parameter to measure target cell DNA interaction with formaldehyde, the data have been, in our opinion, overinterpreted . . . The use of these data for risk assessment purposes is, in our opinion, premature."[57] In contrast, the authors of the paper concluded:

We obviously disagree with . . . [Cohn and coworkers'] opinion. We are in full agreement with Squire and Cameron (1984), who stated that risk assessment should take into consideration all of the available biological data. Squire and Cameron conclude their article on formaldehyde risk assessment with the following remarks: "Evidence presently available on formaldehyde carcinogenic risk generally supports a threshold. At the least, an assumption of nonlinearity at low exposure levels is warranted . . . The use of any risk assessment procedures which fail to incorporate such evidence should explicitly describe . . . the likely overestimates of risk."[58]

Dose: Concentration or Amount?

So far we have considered a variety of arguments about whether the existing experimental data exhibit thresholds or nonlinearities in their dose-response function and whether such behavior is biologically plausible. But in such discussions and in discussions of the epidemiologic results, we need to have a concept of "dose." This is also very important for regulatory policy because it matters a great deal whether one tries to control peak exposures or average exposures. Should we measure dose in terms of concentration or in terms of cumulative amount? In one of the experiments discussed above, the researchers asked: Do the irritant effects of formaldehyde, as measured by increased cell proliferation, depend upon the concentration inhaled or on the amount? In other words, is 3 ppm given for twelve hours equivalent to 12 ppm for three hours? Their results suggested that the concentration of formaldehyde was more decisive—that 12 ppm for three hours was much more damaging than was 3 ppm for twelve hours.[59] Previous work had shown much more toxicity in rats exposed to 15 ppm for six hours a day, five days a week (a total of 450 ppm-hours/week) than in those exposed to 3 ppm of formaldehyde for twenty-two hours a day, seven days a week (462 ppm-hours/week).

As one might expect for irritation, some evidence favors concentration as the more important dose parameter. But it is not known how the *carcinogenic* effects of formaldehyde depend upon concentration, that is, whether the same total amount of formaldehyde given over either shorter or longer periods would yield different frequencies of tumors. For other chemicals the evidence is mixed. In the case of vinyl chloride, peak exposures of short duration appear to be most carcinogenic to humans,[60] but in laboratory animals long-term exposures to low levels are much more tumorigenic than brief exposures to peak levels.[61] Given the strong correlation between the irritant and the carcinogenic properties of formaldehyde, many scientists would predict a relatively greater carcinogenic potential for peak exposures of short duration relative to low-level exposures for longer periods. We return to this issue and consider its implications for quantitative risk assessment in Chapter 6.

Site Specificity

Another issue on which some disagreement exists and which is of special interest to epidemiology concerns the apparent site specificity of formaldehyde—the fact that in rodents formaldehyde causes tumors in the nasal cavity and nowhere else. What about humans? Among those exposed to formaldehyde, should one expect to find tumors in only the nasal cavity; in the nasal cavity, lung, and upper respiratory tract; or in any organ?

Some observers argue for the last possibility on the grounds that many, perhaps most, carcinogens are site specific (or predominant) for different sites in different species, especially species as different as rats and humans. Therefore, although in rodents only squamous cell carcinomas of the nasal cavity were evidently induced by formaldehyde, it is not appropriate to assume that only the nose or only the nose and lungs are possible targets for formaldehyde-induced cancers in humans.

Others point out that most of the formaldehyde that a rat inhales reacts rapidly with, and is absorbed at, the nasal epithelium. This suggests that the toxic effects of formaldehyde are restricted to immediately exposed surfaces, such as the nasal cavity and upper respiratory tract. In experimental dogs most of the inhaled formaldehyde is absorbed before it reaches the lungs.[62] Humans, however, may be exposed to particulate-absorbed formaldehyde or may differ sufficiently in respiratory anatomy or physiology that direct exposure to the lungs themselves is plausible.

Those who argue that formaldehyde is site specific point out that a carcinogen can be "organ specific" in its action in two basic ways. The first is by way of the intrinsic biochemical properties of the compound, the organ site, and the animal species, such that no matter what route is used for dosing—inhalation, ingestion, or injection—tumors arise only in a specific organ or site. For example, certain nitrosamines give rise almost exclusively to tumors of the esophagus, although essentially all other sites of the body are exposed. Similarly, in some species many compounds are tumorigenic only to the liver.

The reasons for this kind of specificity are not well understood, though metabolism is thought to play a decisive role. Most carcinogens are not carcinogens per se, but are actually "precarcinogens" that must be altered by the animal's metabolic processes into an actively carcinogenic form. Because much of an animal's metabolism takes place in the liver, some carcinogens are activated there and go on to form tumors of the liver. Other carcinogens are activated either by a different mechanism (for example, by the resident microorganisms of the intestinal tract) or at different rates or by different kinds of metabolic products, such that organs like the colon or the bladder become targets for tumorigenesis. Since animal species vary in how they process substances, a given compound can easily be specific for one organ in one species and specific for a different organ or organs in another species.

The second way in which a carcinogen may be site-specific depends essentially upon the compound itself. Compounds of this type are carcinogenic in and of themselves: they do not require metabolic activation and instead are considered to be direct-acting. These carcinogens are site specific in that they cause tumors at the first site they hit: the skin, if exposure is to the skin, the mouth and upper gastrointestinal tract if exposure occurs through ingestion, the upper respiratory tract and lungs if exposure is by inhalation, and so on. In general, one would not expect much variation among species in the targets. Tumors would arise only at or very near directly exposed body surfaces.

Formaldehyde appears to be a direct-acting carcinogen. Metabolism appears to *deactivate* it, by oxidizing it to the apparently noncarcinogenic formic acid (or formate). It has been shown, for example, that rats injected with formaldehyde in aqueous solution (formalin) develop tumors at the site of the injection, while rats injected with formic acid develop no such tumors.[63] Similarly, one of six rabbits exposed to formalin by direct application to the palate developed a tumor at that site.[64] Furthermore, formaldehyde is also a direct-acting *mutagen;* it does not require metabolic activation for mutagenicity.

Some analysts argue that this combined evidence makes it reasonable to suspect that people who inhale formaldehyde will develop tumors only in the upper respiratory tract and lungs (and only on the skin and exposed epithelium for people with dermal contact). Critics of this conclusion argue that too little is known about how formaldehyde causes cancer to warrant excluding other organs or sites. They contend that although the major metabolite of formaldehyde is the relatively innocuous formate, it is not the only metabolite. Not all are known, and it is possible that some "metabolized" formaldehyde might be more properly considered "bound" formaldehyde, transported throughout the body and capable of being regenerated in a free and possibly carcinogenic form at various sites.

There is no direct evidence in support of this hypothesis, but there is little data to contradict it. We do know that for many other chemical carcinogens, it is not the major metabolites but the minor ones that cause cancer. Aflatoxin, for example, is a potent liver carcinogen in animals, but when given orally most of the dose is not absorbed into the bloodstream. Only about 1 percent of a dose of aflatoxin is involved in the critical reactions with liver DNA.[65] In general, metabolites are very chemically reactive; otherwise they could not alter DNA. But cellular DNA is much less available for reaction than water, proteins, and other physiological substrates. The result is that carcinogenic interactions between a metabolite and DNA inevitably involve only small fractions of a compound. Hence, the nature of these interactions may or may not be predictable, from knowledge of the major metabolic products.

Summary of Bioassay Issues

It seems clear that at the theoretical and experimental level, most of the critical issues concerning carcinogenesis caused by formaldehyde remain unresolved. The dose-response function in rodents appears to deviate markedly from the idealized straight line through the origin, but there is no agreement about whether the function has a threshold. Arguments about the delivered dose, the mucus blanket, irritation, and endogenous formaldehyde have all been used to suggest that very low levels of formaldehyde are infinitesimally risky. But in each case the evidence, at least in the eyes of some investigators, is ambiguous or inconclusive. Equally important, the evidence from experimental studies cannot provide clear instructions to epidemiologists about the important measures of and expected responses to exposures to formaldehyde. We turn now to the evidence from epidemiological investigations and consider the issues and debates they have engendered.

• Epidemiology and Formaldehyde

From a scientific point of view, the epidemiological findings on formaldehyde and cancer are scant. This is difficult to discern from many of the debates about policy, where these limited findings have assumed a central role. In this section we try to account for some of the differences in the interpretations of and credence ascribed to the results of the epidemiological studies.

The difficulties surrounding their interpretation are not unusual for such studies. Some of the studies were not explicitly designed to examine formaldehyde or any other chemical, but rather to measure the risks associated with a specific occupation. In these studies we know that formaldehyde was involved in the occupational processes studied, but we lack other crucial information. The percentages of study subjects (or control subjects) actually exposed to formaldehyde, the levels of exposure (averages and peaks), the time frames, and combinations with other chemicals, are essentially unknown. Even subjects' cigarette smoking habits are unknown in most studies. This is an important drawback both because the lung is a possible target for formaldehyde-induced cancer and because cigarette smoke itself contains formaldehyde. Reliable assessments of exposure would seem to be crucial to determining that a persuasive link exists between formaldehyde and disease, but such assessments are difficult to attain and have not been developed in even the most recent epidemiology focusing explicitly on formaldehyde.

The details of the epidemiological studies on formaldehyde and cancer have been reviewed elsewhere.[66] Virtually all analysts have come to certain general conclusions, as follows:

- Exposures to formaldehyde have not resulted in detectable increases in deaths from lung cancer, but small increases would not have been detected and therefore cannot be ruled out.

- Formaldehyde exposures have not resulted in detectable increases in deaths from nasal cancer—with some recent exceptions—but even several-fold increases in this risk would not have been detected in the cohort studies conducted to date.

- Small but statistically significant increases in deaths from brain cancer and leukemia have appeared in three different studies of pathologists, anatomists, and embalmers.

We begin by looking at the epidemiologic issues in the three areas of greatest interest: lung cancer, nasal cancer, and, surprisingly, brain cancer and leukemia.

Lung Cancer

If formaldehyde gas is carcinogenic in humans, the most biologically plausible site for its action is the respiratory system. But if one analyzes the lung cancer deaths in all of the epidemiological studies, a somewhat curious result emerges. Three studies found that subjects exposed to formaldehyde had a statistically significant *decrease* in deaths from respiratory system cancer, and six others showed decreases that failed to reach statistical significance.

Analysts are uncertain how to explain this. Some suggest that workers exposed to formaldehyde—pathologists and embalmers, as well as factory workers—might find it uncomfortable or unappealing to smoke cigarettes and in so abstaining are protecting themselves from the biggest cause of lung cancer. Clearly if formaldehyde-exposed individuals smoked markedly less than average, they would have a decreased risk of lung cancer even if formaldehyde was a real, but less potent, lung carcinogen. There are essentially no data, however, on whether formaldehyde-exposed workers actually do smoke less (or more) than expected.

Critics of this line of reasoning consider it unreasonable speculation in the absence of data. Others simply state that the smoking data ought to be collected in the course of the epidemiological studies. A coinvestigator on the large National Cancer Institute (NCI) study on formaldehyde has noted that it is in fact quite difficult to reconstruct such information in studies based primarily upon the review of death certificates and medical records.[67]

One epidemiological study has shown some excess risk of lung cancer among workers at a British industrial plastics factory who were exposed to formaldehyde.[68] The number of deaths from lung cancer among these workers was statistically significant when compared to a national standard, but statistically nonsignificant when compared to the local county standard. The investigators tend to regard the excess lung cancers as ascribable to chance rather than to formaldehyde, but others are not so sure.[69] Overall, though, almost no one believes that the epidemiologic studies completed to date clearly implicate formaldehyde as a cause of lung cancer.

Occupational exposures aside, some point to the possibility that formaldehyde in cigarette smoke is partially responsible for lung disease and cancer.[70] There are certainly parallels between lung carcinogenesis in humans caused by cigarette smoke and nasal carcinogenesis in rats caused by formaldehyde. Both processes involve chronic irritation, followed by squamous cell metaplasia, followed by squamous cell carcinoma. Furthermore, in one study in which mice were exposed to gaseous formaldehyde, their respiratory tracts also exhibited many of the dose-dependent changes observed in the epithelia of smokers' lungs: hyperplasia, stratification, metaplasia, and dysplasia.[71]

The link between the formaldehyde content of cigarette smoke and its carcinogenicity is difficult to forge, primarily because smoke contains several other irritants and many other known or suspected carcinogens.[72] The special legal and regulatory status of cigarettes also places the issue outside of the formaldehyde policy debates.

Nonetheless, some analysts consider it deceptive to discuss "the formaldehyde problem" without some reference to this highest—and conceivably most hazardous—source of human exposure.

Nasal Cancer

The human nose is also a likely target for formaldehyde gas, but until very recently no increases in the death rate from nasal cancer had been detected in any epidemiologic studies. John Higginson, former director of IARC, believes that the epidemiological evidence is sufficient to exclude formaldehyde from serious consideration as a significant nasal carcinogen in humans. In 1982 in a letter to the chairwoman of the CPSC, Nancy Stoerts, he wrote: "The type of cancer one might believe to be produced by formaldehyde gas is normally rare. Any marked excess should be easy to recognize in view of the large scale on which the chemical has been used for many years."[73]

Many other analysts point to the difficulty of detecting even sizable increases in risk for such rare diseases as nasal cancer. The Federal Panel on Formaldehyde, for example, wrote: "The major difficulty of the mortality studies of individuals exposed to formaldehyde is the limited ability of such studies to detect excess risk for rare causes of death. Since the known carcinogenic action of formaldehyde is limited to the nasal sinuses in rats, there is a need to evaluate the risk for this site in man . . . It is unlikely that a cohort of sufficient size can be assembled to accomplish this task."[74]

The authors of a large occupational cohort study designed to investigate formaldehyde, who are generally inclined to agree with Higginson, nonetheless agree with the federal panel on this point. They examined a cohort of 7,680 men, of whom 1,626 had died. None of the deaths were caused by nasal cancer. But because of the rarity of the disease, only 1.07 such deaths would have been expected. The authors calculated that even a study the size of theirs had only "an even chance of detecting a relative risk of 5 . . . Under more conservative assumptions . . . there is only a slightly better than even chance of having detected a 10-fold increase in risk."[75] The authors mentioned some eleven other studies that were negative for excess nasal cancer among those occupationally exposed to formaldehyde, but their appreciation of the limits of these studies led them to conclude that "it is premature to rule out a carcinogenic action of formaldehyde at this site.[76]

Higginson agrees that all the "data taken together are insufficient to completely exclude a minimal risk," but also adds that "certainly they weigh heavily against the view that formaldehyde gas constitutes any considerable risk for nasal cancer to man."[77] Higginson does not appear to have considered sites other than the nasal cavity with respect to formaldehyde's possible carcinogenicity.

The Federal Panel on Formaldehyde and others have suggested that case-control studies of nasal cancer would be more powerful than the more typical cohort studies as a way of investigating this question. A case-control study starts by gathering a group of individuals with nasal cancer and a group of suitably matched controls who do not have nasal cancer. Then analysts try to determine whether the cancer patients were more likely than the controls to have been exposed to formaldehyde or other putative carcinogens. Nasal carcinoma has in fact been investigated in several case-control studies. Results of all but the most recent studies did not indicate that patients with nasal cancer had sustained unusual exposures to formaldehyde. One set of investigators did find that work in the textile industry appeared to be a "potentially important occupation" for the development of nasal cancer.[78] Few analysts were willing to judge, however, whether the cancer was caused by textile dust, formaldehyde, or chance. The majority felt that the definitive case-control study for nasal cancer and formaldehyde had yet to be performed.

A group of researchers in Denmark has reported positive results from their case-control study of nasal cancer.[79] The study represented the first attempt to link the data in the Danish Cancer Registry to the employment data recorded by the national pension fund. The case group of 488 consisted of all those diagnosed as having carcinoma of the nasal cavity or sinuses any time from 1970 to 1982. Controls were patients with cancers at unrelated sites, matched for sex, age, and year of diagnosis.

The results were that males with a history of occupational exposure to formaldehyde had a statistically significant ($p < 0.05$) elevated risk for nasal cancer. Their relative risk was 2.8, with a 95 percent confidence interval of 1.8 to 4.3. Exposures to wood dust—an established nasal tumorigen—and to paint, lacquer, and glue carried relative risks of 2.5 and 2.1, respectively. Exposure to both wood dust and formaldehyde appeared to be additive in increasing a worker's relative risk of nasal cancer. Wood dust also confounds the results, however. When one adjusts for it by standard techniques, the relative risk for formaldehyde exposure alone is reduced to 1.6. The authors state that this relative risk "is not significantly in excess of 1.0, although still compatible with a 3- to 4-fold increase in risk using conventional 95 percent confidence limits." That is, even if the true relative risk is 3 or 4, there is a 5 percent chance that the relative risk would *appear* as small as that which was observed.

This is exactly the kind of result that admits to opposing interpretations. Maybe the excess risk associated with formaldehyde is apparent but not real, caused only by wood dust. Maybe it is quite real but too small to be convincingly demonstrated by this single study. Only five males with nasal cancer in the study had been both exposed to formaldehyde and not exposed to wood dust.

The authors tend to consider their results positive, having titled their report "Occupational Formaldehyde Exposure and Increased Nasal Cancer Risk in Man." They write that "none of the relative risk estimates among women are significantly increased"—perhaps because only about half as many women as men were in the study group—but add that "it is worth noting that the risks in relation to formaldehyde (RR = 2.8) and paint, lacquer and glue (RR = 1.9) are at the same level as among males." They term their work "the first study to indicate that formaldehyde exposure may lead to a slight but statistically significant increase in nasal cancer risk for humans." And finally, they write that "if causal, some 7% of all cases of nasal carcinoma among men in Denmark can be attributed to occupational formaldehyde exposure."

Brain Cancer and Leukemia

The situation for brain cancer and leukemia is in some senses the reverse of that for lung and nasal cancer. Although respiratory system cancers caused by formaldehyde are biologically plausible, the numbers have not appeared to be in excess in most of the epidemiological investigations. For brain cancer and leukemia, it is difficult to construct a biologically plausible mechanism for formaldehyde-induced effects, but epidemiological investigations have repeatedly revealed excesses of these cancers among *some* occupationally exposed groups.

The difficulty in constructing a plausible mechanism stems from the rapid chemical reactivity of formaldehyde. Some investigators have shown that when a dose of formaldehyde is inhaled, most of it reacts with the nasal epithelium, leaving less than 1 percent to be deposited in the brain, bone marrow, or other distant sites.[80] Others have also shown that the biological half-life for formaldehyde in the circulation is only 1.5 minutes.[81] This means that the amount that does reach the brain or bone marrow is likely to have been oxidized into formate or otherwise metabolized rather than be in its original reactive form.

Five epidemiological studies have been made of pathologists, anatomists, and embalmers. The risk of brain cancer was significantly elevated in three of these studies and slightly elevated in the other two. Leukemia risk also appeared to be significantly elevated in three and slightly elevated in two. The excess risks are not very large, but their appearance within these medical cohorts was sufficiently regular and statistically significant to cause concern among some analysts.

Few know how to account for the results. The findings appear too consistent to be the result of chance. These individuals are occupationally exposed to other volatile chemicals in embalming and fixative solutions, but no one seriously suspects that these other chemicals are any more to blame than formaldehyde. The Epidemiology Panel of the Formaldehyde Consensus Conference, after considering the findings on brain cancer and leukemia, decided that it was not possible to implicate formaldehyde causally from these studies. But the panel stated: "Aside from formaldehyde and human tissue, however, it is unclear what other important occupational exposures these professional groups shared."[82]

Some epidemiologists have argued that the studies may be biased in one respect. They note that some brain tumors are difficult to diagnose except upon autopsy. An unusually high proportion of medical professionals undergo autopsy, and therefore it appears that they die of brain cancer more than others do, even in the absence of any real excess risk. In one epidemiological study that explicitly adjusted for this "diagnostic sensitivity" bias in selecting its control populations, however, the excess risk of brain cancer remained.[83] Furthermore, other epidemiologists recognize no such bias. In discussing the results of their study of British pathologists, which showed an excess of deaths from brain tumors, researchers wrote: "It is difficult to decide what, apart from chance, might be the possible cause of the excess deaths from brain cancer in this population. Social class gradients are relatively unimportant in this tumor, neither is there an excess among medical practitioners as a group."[84]

None of the epidemiological studies on formaldehyde-exposed factory workers—as opposed to medical professionals—reveals excess risks of either brain cancer or leukemia. Some analysts reason that if both groups are exposed to formaldehyde, but only one group develops excess brain cancers and leukemia, then it is unreasonable to hold formaldehyde responsible. Others argue that the excess risk among the professional groups appears to be real and that this does not necessarily implicate formaldehyde, but until a more plausible explanation is forthcoming, formaldehyde should remain under suspicion.

Overall Views

Most analysts agree that no firm conclusions can yet be drawn from the existing epidemiological studies. But there are serious differences of interpretation and emphasis. Some suggest that the results really mean that formaldehyde is unlikely to cause human cancer, some are truly neutral on the subject, and still others read the results to mean there is a real probability that formaldehyde is a human carcinogen.

Not surprisingly, the middle position is the most popular. A working group of IARC, for example, having reviewed the epidemiological reports published through 1981, concluded that no conclusions could be drawn: "The epidemiological studies provide inadequate evidence to assess the carcinogenicity of formaldehyde in man."[85]

In contrast, the EPA under Gorsuch tended to view the epidemiological studies as having exonerated formaldehyde. "Three epidemiology studies presented at CIIT are in agreement that there is no excess in nasal or respiratory cancer or even a significant increase in any form of cancer which could be attributed to formaldehyde. Although the individual studies may be limited in scope, when combined they clearly indicate no increased risk in the exposed population."[86] Others who share this view maintain it is very unlikely that the excess cancers that have appeared among some formaldehyde-exposed cohorts were caused by formaldehyde. Lawyers for the Formaldehyde Institute noted that neither epidemiological studies nor any other data conclusively prove the negative (that there is no cancer risk whatsoever), but also wrote: "No epidemiologic study has attributed any nasal or other cancer to formaldehyde . . . The fact that formaldehyde has been used for decades (at levels significantly higher than today) with no evidence of cancer in humans is a common sense indication that no significant risk is present."[87]

In contrast, two representatives of the NRDC move a bit away from neutrality in the opposite direction: "Epidemiologic studies completed to date . . . have been inconclusive or suggestive of a positive

effect rather than negative regarding the carcinogenicity of formaldehyde . . . A number of studies have been suggestive of an increased
cancer risk . . . Recently there have been several reports of rare nasal
tumors in workers exposed to formaldehyde."[88]

Scientists who believe that the epidemiological findings on formaldehyde have turned up nothing do tend to differ, in the certainty
with which they state it, from nonscientists who share that belief.
John Higginson may be foremost among the scientists who believe
that exposure to formaldehyde does not constitute a carcinogenic
risk. But even after citing a large number of negative epidemiological
studies in support of this position, he adds: "All these data taken
together are insufficient to completely exclude a minimal risk."[89]
Perhaps Higginson realizes that the power of all these epidemiological studies is limited and that if some future study did implicate
formaldehyde, this would not be inconsistent with the negative results to date.

The epidemiologists themselves are reluctant to draw conclusions
from their own work. Investigators from The Medical Research Council (MRC), for example, conducted the largest study to date specifically designed to investigate formaldehyde. With the possible
exception of some increases in lung cancer deaths at one of six plants
investigated, the results appeared to be quite negative. The report
stated: "The findings of this study do not support the hypothesis that
formaldehyde is a human carcinogen."[90] But they immediately added:
"The strength of the negative evidence is, however, limited by the
small number of men (605) exposed to "high" levels for more than 5
years and followed for more than 20 years after first exposure. Further
studies of groups exposed to formaldehyde are needed."[91]

The editorial writers of the British medical journal *The Lancet*, in
contrast, draw more from the results of that study. They briefly
presented the data, then concluded: "No doubt all these data will be
exhaustively analyzed over the next couple of years, and conclusions
will be hedged about with the usual cautious provisions. However, it
seems very unlikely that occupational formaldehyde exposures prevalent today will be carrying any risk of cancer and it would be unreasonable for the IARC working group, were it to reconvene with the
full MRC data before it, to find the epidemiological data still
'inadequate.' "[92]

These differences in tone are not surprising. Faced with less than
decisive evidence, working scientists are inclined to conclude that
more research is needed. Editorial writers and lawyers are inclined to

weigh the evidence at hand and form a judgment. By training and circumstance they have quite different views about the urgency of reaching a decision versus the appropriateness of caution or neutrality in the face of ambiguous evidence.

Implications of Ongoing Studies

The National Cancer Institute has recently completed a study of some 26,000 workers exposed to formaldehyde.[93] As shown in Table 3.3, no excess mortality from specific cancers or overall cancer appeared. What can we learn from these apparently negative results? To what extent can we say that these findings from the NCI study contradict the CIIT bioassay results?

Some argue that such a result casts doubt upon the fidelity of rat models for human situations, that rats must be much more sensitive to formaldehyde's effects than humans. Careful examination and extrapolation of the bioassay data, however, reveal that even if humans and rats are equally susceptible to formaldehyde-induced cancer, negative results are not unexpected. This is because at the levels of formaldehyde experienced by workers, the cancer risk predicted from the CIIT bioassay data is in a peculiar range. Although the risk is often judged too large to be dismissed as insignificant for purposes of regulatory policy, it may be too small to be detected even by an epidemiological investigation of 26,000 workers. To clarify this point, we will discuss a few aspects of one of EPA's risk assessments of formaldehyde. Details of these predictions are debatable—as we consider in depth in Chapter 6—but they allow us to show how "significant" risks may not be observable.

We start with a conservative assumption, namely that the exposures to formaldehyde of the 26,000 workers, and hence their risks, are equivalent to those of apparel manufacturers exposed to an average of 1 ppm. (This assumption overestimates the cohort's actual exposure and risk.) EPA's estimate for lifetime cancer risk for apparel workers is that for every 100,000 workers, 2 more will die of cancer than would have without this occupational formaldehyde exposure. Clearly, then, even if every one of the 26,000 workers were followed until his death, the additional one-half death from cancer would not be detectable. A study of 26,000 workers is not, however, a study of 26,000 deaths: only 3,268 had died by the study's end. Among these 3,268, then, one might expect—but of course could not observe—only an additional 0.1 cancer death.

Table 3.3 Cancer mortality among white male industrial workers exposed to formaldehyde.

Cause	Observed	Expected	SMR[a]	95 percent CI[b] (SMR)
All cancers				
Exposed (>0.1 ppm)	570	566	101	83–109
Unexposed (<0.1 ppm)	158	168	94	80–110
Skin				
Exposed	10	12	80	38–147
Unexposed	2	3	—	—
Lung				
Exposed	201	182	111	96–127
Unexposed	49	53	93	69–123
Nose				
Exposed	2	2.2	—	—
Unexposed	0	0.6	—	—
Larynx				
Exposed	12	8	142	73–248
Unexposed	4	3	—	—
Buccal cavity and pharynx				
Exposed	18	19	96	57–152
Unexposed	3	6	54	11–157
Brain and CNS				
Exposed	17	21	81	47–130
Unexposed	6	6	102	38–223
Leukemia				
Exposed	19	24	80	48–124
Unexposed	4	7	58	16–148

Source: A. Blair et al., "Mortality among Industrial Workers Exposed to Formaldehyde," *Journal of the National Cancer Institute,* 76 (1986): 1071–1084.

a. SMR = standardized mortality ratio (ratio of observed to expected deaths multiplied by 100). The SMR is not given when observed and expected numbers are less than 5.

b. CI = confidence interval.

Even EPA's upper 95 percent confidence limit of the estimated risk—5.5×10^{-4}—amounts to only about 3 more deaths from cancer among the deaths of 5,000 workers exposed to formaldehyde. If these deaths were caused by lung cancer, the excess would fall far short of statistical significance. About 250 lung cancer deaths would be expected among 3,268 deaths in any event, so 253 such deaths would not be statistically significantly higher. If the excess deaths were all nasal cancer deaths, however, the power of the epidemiology would be increased somewhat. Because this is such a rare cancer, only about two nasal cancer deaths would be expected in the absence of excess risk, but about four would be observed if formaldehyde was carcinogenic as predicted. But the estimate of two excess nasal cancer deaths is likely to be an overestimate. It derives, as noted, from the upper 95 percent confidence limit of the estimate range, and the exposure patterns for apparel workers put them at greater predicted risk than the exposure patterns for most of the other occupations that were investigated.

These calculations illustrate that even a study this large has little power to detect the predicted excesses in cancer deaths. Hence, in retrospect the negative results of the other, smaller, epidemiologic studies are not surprising. The predicted risks for formaldehyde are too small to be detected by even very large epidemiological studies. This is not to make the policy judgment that these risks should or should not be reduced through regulation. It is only to say that any estimates of such risks cannot be either supported or refuted by epidemiological investigations.

• Mutagenicity Tests and In Vitro Mechanisms

A third source of data on the effects of formaldehyde is provided by studies of its mutagenic effects in animals and in cells in culture. In some ways, though, these data are even more difficult to interpret for policy purposes than those already reviewed.

Long before it was a subject of regulatory debate, formaldehyde was a topic of study in mutation research. Studies in the late 1940s revealed that the larvae of *Drosophila* (fruit flies) mutate when reared on food spiked with formaldehyde.[94] The results of these and other experiments raised quite a few questions. For example, it appeared that only male larvae mutate under these conditions. Female larvae do not, nor do adult *Drosophila* of either sex. The dose-response relationships were not what researchers expected. In some cases mutagenicity showed no dependence upon dose over a several-fold range, and in other studies the toxicity of the formaldehyde-treated food was inversely related to its mutagenicity. Positive but often weak and "nonclassical" results from mutagenicity studies on various other species led to many different hypotheses about the mechanisms of formaldehyde's genetic and cytological effects. It now seems likely that no single hypothesis will prove to be "correct," primarily because formaldehyde reacts rapidly and nonselectively and because it has been evaluated under many different systems.[95]

In interpreting these research results, it is important to distinguish between mutagenicity studies and mutagenicity tests. Although the two overlap somewhat, the studies tend to be performed primarily for scientific purposes, while the tests are conducted primarily to inform policy decisions. Scientists study the mutagenicity of a given chemical in *Drosophila*, for example, to probe the mechanisms of mutagenicity, whether or not humans are exposed to the chemical. In contrast, the mutagenicity of a given chemical is tested in standard assays such as the Ames assay, for example, precisely because humans are exposed to the chemical and because one wishes to learn something of its mutagenic and carcinogenic risk for regulatory purposes. It is therefore no surprise that combining the results of the many studies and the many tests on formaldehyde to "assess" its mutagenicity is highly problematic. The studies and tests have been done not only on different organisms, under different conditions, and to measure different end points; they have been done for fundamentally different reasons.

From a policy perspective, there are several reasons to test a chemical for mutagenicity. One is to determine quickly and inexpensively, by means of a short-term test such as the Ames assay, whether a new compound (one on which there is little information about its chronic toxicity) is mutagenic or otherwise damaging to DNA. If it is, this is taken to signal its potential for inducing cancer in animals. In other words, one uses these tests as screens, and positive results warn the observer of the likelihood of other adverse effects. Interestingly, though, results of such tests are not always easily interpreted. The question "Is it a mutagen?" can be as overly simplistic and difficult to answer responsibly as the question "Is it a carcinogen?"

Such is the case for formaldehyde. The compound is very reactive and volatile—it is, after all, a gas at room temperature. In most mutagenicity tests, however, incubations are at temperatures higher than room temperature. As a result, investigators can easily lose much or all of a given amount of formaldehyde in the very act of attempting to assay it. Early results with the Ames assay, for example, were negative.[96] A slight modification of the assay revealed that formaldehyde was "very weak[ly]" mutagenic.[97] A more extensively modified Ames assay and the use of a new Ames tester strain[98] more plainly showed formaldehyde to be mutagenic. Given the various mutagenicity tests, one report concluded: "In reviewing the . . . literature, we have found that the recent work is more likely to find formaldehyde a mutagen than earlier studies and is also more likely to show a dose-response relationship."[99]

Given the results of the CIIT carcinogenicity study in rats and mice, one could use these mutagenicity tests to, as OSHA puts it, "confirm results provided by animal bioassays."[100] OSHA states that "'the probability of a false-positive result for a chemical which is positive in one well-conducted bioassay and one well-validated short-term test is extremely small."[101] Some researchers seem to go even further, at least as a matter of generic policy. Leon Golberg, former president of CIIT, writes: "Positive results in several, valid short-term tests indicate that, without waiting for the results of long-term animal exposure studies, operations involving the chemical should be immediately examined and human exposure reduced to as far as is practicable."[102]

Although formaldehyde does show positive results in several short-term mutagenicity tests, many scientists are nonetheless not convinced that it is a potential carcinogen at typical levels of exposure. Thus, despite generic cancer guidelines, most scientists are not willing to be bound by such decision rules and instead tend to form more ad hoc judgments on a chemical-by-chemical basis.

A third reason to perform short-term tests is to learn more about the mechanisms of interaction between the compound or its metabolites and the genetic material. Some compounds, for example, appear to be carcinogenic without mutagenizing or otherwise perceptibly damaging DNA. Many of these have been termed tumor promoters—as was explained in the case of turpentine's effect on mouse skin—as opposed to tumor initiators. Some analysts, as we noted above, maintained at least initially that formaldehyde appeared to be a tumor promoter (acting through its irritating effect) and as such was unlikely to be carcinogenic at very low doses. This claim, however, was not consistent with all of the experimental evidence. Although high doses of formaldehyde do resemble some tumor promoters in causing cytotoxicity and hyperplasia, formaldehyde is also plainly genotoxic. Formaldehyde covalently alters DNA, cross-linking strands of DNA both to other DNA and to proteins. Formaldehyde is demonstrably mutagenic in *Drosophila*, yeast, fungi, some bacteria, and cultured mammalian cells, including cells from humans.

Once a compound is shown to be a mutagen, it is tempting to try to determine its mutagenic potency. This topic gave the panel of the Consensus Workshop on Formaldehyde a good deal of trouble. The scientists just asked one another, "Well, what do you mean, how strong is it?" In general, of course, the question has some meaning. A compound such as methylnitronitrosoguanidine (MNNG), which generates lots of mutants from a relatively small amount of compound relative to other substances that have been tested, is certainly a strong mutagen, at least in a particular test system under a particular set of conditions. But there are no scientifically defined categories of strong mutagen, moderately strong mutagen, moderately weak mutagen, and so on, especially when the results of many different test systems are somehow to be assimilated.

The Consensus Workshop panel concluded, "The data we have reviewed are consistent with formaldehyde acting as a weak mutagen (i.e., less than 10-fold increase over background)."[103] But it is important to recognize that "10-fold" was only and could only be a very rough and unmethodically figured average, and that there is no a priori basis for deciding to use such a figure to distinguish weak mutagens. In fact, there was considerable discussion about whether formaldehyde might be better classified as a moderately weak or weak-to-moderate mutagen. Furthermore, and central to our purposes, is the realization that such a scientifically empty terminological discussion would have been of very little interest in the absence of impending policy decisions. Characterizing the strength of mutagenic activity in a way that is consistent and coherent across compounds is not a problem that biologists would find particularly relevant or interesting if they were setting their own agenda for purely scientific purposes.

A fourth reason to test mutagenicity is to determine whether people exposed to the chemical might produce offspring with genetic defects. Lacking epidemiological evidence on formaldehyde as a cause of birth defects, one might nonetheless suspect the chemical of contributing to heritable disease if it mutagenized the sperm or eggs of laboratory animals. Formaldehyde does not appear to have this ability, although it has not been extensively tested in this regard. Overall, neither genetic effects nor mechanisms of mutagenesis have been central to the science-policy debates on formaldehyde.

• Conclusion

Having reviewed the difficult scientific debates about formaldehyde, we find it easier to understand why regulatory decision makers have differed in what they make of formaldehyde. In summary:

The animal studies show clear evidence of carcinogenicity at some doses. The dose-response function in the experimental range appears to be quite nonlinear for malignant tumors induced in rats. No malignant tumors appeared in the animals exposed to the lowest doses.

Scientists continue to dispute the probable magnitude of risk at low doses. Some believe that either a no-effect threshold exists or that very small doses pose vanishingly small risks. Such views are based in part on the nonlinear dose-response curve in rodents and on some evidence that cytotoxic and genotoxic responses are attenuated at very low levels of exposure. Others doubt the biological relevance of much of the mechanistic research on formaldehyde carcinogenesis and believe there is probably no threshold in the dose-response function. These scientists and others believe that formaldehyde—like all carcinogens—should be "presumed" to present an excess cancer risk at any dose in order to err on the side of safety. This debate has become entangled with a more general debate about the use of mechanistic information in policy setting, which in turn seems clearly influenced by policy advocacy and strategic concerns.

Observers disagree about the seriousness of positive epidemiological results for tumors and sites that are not easy to explain, given what is known about the compound's behavior in the human body. The positive results for brain tumors and the lower-than-expected lung cancer rates make the overall interpretation of the epidemiology problematic.

Given the limited carcinogenic potency of low levels of formaldehyde in rodents, cohort studies of humans exposed to formaldehyde may have to be impossibly large to reveal any excess cancers. The majority opinion seems to be that the existing epidemiology is not very informative. Nonetheless, some advocates have been willing to read (contradictory) substantive results into the available findings.

Although formaldehyde has often been positive in mutagenicity tests, it is not easy to use this information to help resolve existing policy disputes, except perhaps to undercut the argument that the compound is only a promoter via irritation.

* * *

It is clear that the scientific debate has been shaped in various ways by the policy process with which it interacts. Many of the questions that have been posed, as well as the answers that have been offered, arise because of pending regulatory actions. Scientifically, formaldehyde is a difficult case. The generic guidelines for uniform cancer policy do not seem to many scientists to fully capture the implications of the pattern of evidence as a whole. Yet as we saw in the last chapter, regulators eager to justify their decisions to the courts and to avoid responsibility before the public have needed to create and rely upon decision rules that at least appear to be "scientific."

The larger question is how regulatory agencies should decide these cases. Should society insist that nondiscretionary rules be used to set regulatory policy, or should attempts be made to use the judgments of working scientists on a case-by-case basis? If we take the latter course, how can we assure political accountability for implicit policy judgments about how to resolve uncertainty? How can regulators recognize the legitimate and critical role of science without promising more than scientists can deliver? These are the issues we return to in Chapters 6 and 7, but first we have another—and very different—case to consider.

4 • THE PROBLEM OF SETTING STANDARDS

ONE OF the most controversial proposals for chemical regulation during the Carter administration was OSHA's unsuccessful attempt to reduce the permissible level of exposure to benzene in the workplace from 10 ppm to 1 ppm. The same issue arose at OSHA during the Reagan administration. The debate about benzene is of particular interest because it raises fundamental questions about the regulation of toxic chemicals.

Like formaldehyde, benzene is a useful industrial chemical. It is recovered commercially largely from petroleum and, to a lesser extent, from coal. In 1980 the United States alone produced more than 5 million tons. World production is perhaps three times that of the United States, making benzene the fourth or fifth largest volume organic chemical on a worldwide basis.[1] Its major use in the past was in blends with gasoline, but this use has been declining in the United States. At one time benzene was also used extensively as a solvent for paints and rubber and in rubber cement, which is widely used in the production of shoes, garments, and artificial leather. Today benzene is employed primarily as a chemical intermediate in the production of other industrial compounds used in making plastics, resins, dyes, and pesticides.

OSHA estimates that approximately 270,000 workers are exposed to benzene in the major industry sectors that fall under the agency's jurisdiction.[2] These sectors include the various benzene producers (petrochemicals, petroleum refining, and coke and chemical manufacturing), manufacturers of rubber tires, and firms engaged in the bulk storage and transportation of benzene or of petroleum products containing benzene. The durations of workers' exposures to benzene are not well defined, but the average concentrations for most exposed workers are in the range of 0 to 1.0 ppm. Relatively few workers are exposed to 10 ppm, but about 25,000 to 30,000 workers receive frequent exposures between 1 and 10 ppm.

EPA has also taken an interest in regulating benzene because the public is exposed to it from automotive exhaust, industrial facilities, and gasoline service stations. Average ambient concentrations of benzene range from 1 to 100 ppm in American cities.[3] In a survey of twelve states, about 300,000 people were estimated to be exposed to benzene in the air from coke ovens, with concentrations usually in the range of several ppb. Benzene concentrations in the air near U.S. chemical manufacturing plants have been recorded between 0.6 and 34 ppb. Finally, the air near gasoline service stations and other fueling facilities contains benzene concentrations anywhere from several ppb to several ppm.

Unlike the case of formaldehyde, concern about benzene-induced carcinogenicity was initially stimulated by clinical case information and epidemiological data rather than by animal bioassay results. Indeed, for many years benzene was considered one of the few known human carcinogens—specifically, a leukemogen—that had not been shown to be carcinogenic to animals. Today benzene is recognized as a carcinogen at several sites in several animal species, even though an adequate animal model of benzene-induced leukemia has not been developed.

The positive human data stimulated regulatory action first at OSHA in the 1970s and later at EPA. The controversy was heated in spite of the positive human data. Scientists disputed dose-response issues while interest groups clashed over what decision rules should be used by regulators.

Although this chapter examines primarily OSHA's benzene rulemaking and to a lesser extent EPA's rulemaking, the underlying policy issues have arisen in many other instances. In fact, the Carter administration's treatment of benzene was a pivotal point in the history of toxic chemical regulation because it stimulated Supreme Court rulings on the proper roles of quantitative risk assessment and cost-benefit analysis in rulemaking.

• Congress and the OSHA Mandate

As recently as the mid-1960s, the case for aggressive federal action on occupational health and safety problems was not widely debated.

The original proposal for a federal initiative on workplace safety was advanced by one of President Lyndon Johnson's speechwriters, not by organized labor or public-health groups. The idea was nurtured by Esther Peterson, one of the assistant secretaries in the Labor Department, who had become concerned about a high incidence of lung cancer among uranium miners. According to Steven Kelman, the idea of a new federal agency for workplace safety is a classic example of "agenda formation" in the political process. Occupational health and safety came before Congress because a few political entrepreneurs were searching for "good causes" during the latter years of the Johnson administration.[4]

Johnson's original legislative proposal went nowhere in 1968. In November 1968, however, a mine disaster in Farmington, West Virginia, took seventy-eight lives. This incident gave emotional impetus to the case for strong legislation on workers' safety and health. In 1969 both the Nixon administration and the Democratic leadership in Congress introduced major bills on these matters. By this time the safety issue had become an important priority for lobbyists of the American Federation of Labor–Congress of Industrial Organizations (AFL-CIO). Moreover, political momentum was building behind "Naderism" and "environmentalism," providing additional support for regulation of unsafe business practices. Concern over industrial accidents rather than long-term health risks played the dominant role in these early political debates.

Passage of the final OSHA bill in 1970 was not accomplished without major points of disagreement and compromise. Nixon's proposal differed from the Democratic proposal over the proper institutional home for the new agency. Republicans and business lobbyists wanted regulatory power to be vested in an independent commission, while Democrats and organized labor wanted the new agency to be part of the Department of Labor. The final version reflected labor's plan, thereby strengthening the notion that OSHA was intended to be an advocate of the health and safety interests of workers rather than an analytical (neutral) balancer of worker and business interests.[5]

The Occupational Safety and Health Act of 1970 places some limitations on OSHA's authority to require safe and healthful working conditions. The agency's major regulatory tool is defined in section 3(8) of the act: "The term 'occupational safety and health standard' means a standard which requires conditions, or the adoption or use of one or more practices, means, methods, operations, or processes, *reasonably necessary or appropriate* to provide safe or healthful employment and places of employment" (emphasis added).[6] The original House and Senate versions of OSHA's statute both contained provisions identical to section 3(8). In the legislative history, however, the phrase "reasonably necessary or appropriate" was not discussed. In the early years of OSHA, section 3(8) was not considered to be a legally significant provision in the context of promulgating permanent health standards.[7]

Concerning toxic materials such as benzene, Congress provided some explicit guidance to OSHA in section 6(b)(5): "The Secretary, in promulgating standards dealing with toxic materials or harmful physical agents, shall set the standard *which most adequately assures, to the extent feasible,* on the basis of the best available evidence, *that no employee will suffer material impairment* of health or functional capacity" (emphasis added).[8]

The history of section 6(b)(5) is complicated. The original House bill, proposed by Representative Domenick Daniels, required the secretary to set a standard "which most adequately assures, on the basis of the best available professional evidence, that no employee will suffer any impairment of health or functional capacity or diminished life expectancy."[9] The original Senate version was identical to the Daniels bill, except for an amendment by Senator Jacob Javits that required the secretary to set the standard "which most adequately and feasibly assures that no employee will suffer any impairment of health."[10] The Javits amendment to the original Senate bill was described as "an improvement over the Daniels bill which might be interpreted to require absolute health and safety in all cases, regardless of feasibility."[11]

On the Senate floor Senator Peter Dominick continued to express concern that the act might be read to require absolute safety.[12] He feared that the secretary might find it feasible to "ban all occupations in which there remains *some* risk of injury, impaired health, or life expectancy."[13] Dominick warned the Senate that section 6(b)(5), if literally applied, could "close every business in this nation."

Although Senator Dominick failed to accomplish his original goal of deleting the first sentence of 6(b)(5), he did persuade Senators Harrison Williams and Javits to support an amended version that became 6(b)(5) as it now appears in the act. The final version limited the applicability of 6(b)(5) to "toxic materials and harmful physical agents," changed "health impairment" to "material impairment of health," and deleted the reference to "diminished life expectancy." Instead of the phrase "which most adequately assures," Dominick substituted "which most adequately assures, to the extent feasible."[14] The House and Senate then overwhelmingly approved the act with Dominick's version of 6(b)(5).[15] These changes proved to be, as we shall see, extremely important in the Supreme Court's rulings on OSHA's authority to regulate toxic chemicals.

• OSHA's First Benzene Rulemaking

One of OSHA's initial actions in the area of health was adoption of a regulation designed to protect workers from the toxic effects of benzene on the blood. In 1971 OSHA adopted a PEL for benzene of 10 ppm measured as an eight-hour TWA. The regulation contains a ceiling exposure of 25 ppm and allowances for brief excursions up to 50 ppm. This PEL, which was not reduced until 1987, was based on a "national consensus standard" developed by the American National Standards Institute (ANSI).[16] At the time the 10 ppm limit was adopted, a lower PEL of 1 ppm was given only brief consideration, perhaps because benzene's ability to induce leukemia, although suspected, was not yet widely appreciated.

During the 1970s a combination of emerging epidemiological evidence and pressure from the United Rubber Workers (URW) caused OSHA to consider stricter benzene regulation as a safeguard against the risk of leukemia. Early petitions by labor leaders were rebuffed by OSHA,[17] even though both NIOSH and a panel of the National Academy of Sciences described benzene as a suspected human leukemogen.[18] The issue began to heat up in 1976 when NIOSH updated its earlier criteria document on benzene and recommended that OSHA lower the benzene exposure standard from 10 to 1 ppm.[19]

Enter Eula Bingham

The election of Jimmy Carter in November 1976 and the appointment of Eula Bingham as OSHA administrator led the agency to take a more activist posture on health issues. Not only was Bingham a scientist with expertise in occupational health, she had a strong reputation as an advocate of workers' rights, and she was the first administrator of OSHA under a Democratic president. The agency had been criticized both for setting many trivial safety standards and for neglecting health issues.[20] Bingham was determined to use her expertise in helping the agency make some new initiatives on controlling toxic chemicals in the workplace.[21]

Benzene had become something of a symbol of regulatory inaction in the area of occupational health standards. Bingham decided to make it her first order of business.[22] Even before her appointment was confirmed by the Senate, she began work on an emergency temporary standard (ETS) for benzene.[23] Her staff and lawyers in the Labor Department pointed out that OSHA had no new scientific evidence to justify such an urgent regulatory move. As we noted in Chapter 2, an ETS must be justified on the basis of "grave danger" to workers.[24] That legal hurdle was to be overcome by prompt completion of a NIOSH study of the effects of benzene exposures on workers at a Goodyear plant in St. Mary's, Ohio. The principal investigator of that study, Peter Infante, was reportedly urged by OSHA officials to publish his results as soon as possible.[25]

On April 28, 1977, Bingham signed a 1 ppm ETS for benzene.[26] That same morning a lawyer for the AFL-CIO submitted a lawsuit to the Circuit Court of Appeals of the District of Columbia (the D.C. Circuit) requesting judicial review of the ETS. Several weeks later the ETS was also challenged in the Fifth Circuit Court of Appeals (New Orleans) by the American Petroleum Institute (API). The ETS was to take effect on May 21, 1977, but on May 20 a judge from the Fifth Circuit issued an interim restraining order preventing OSHA from implementing and enforcing the ETS.

Although the OSHA statute directs that judicial reviews should take place in the court where a challenge is first filed,[27] petroleum industry petitioners urged the D.C. Circuit to return the case to the Fifth Circuit on the grounds that the AFL-CIO lawsuit had been filed prematurely. In a two-to-one decision, the D.C. Circuit held that the interests of justice demanded transferring the case to the Fifth Circuit for disposition.[28] This "court shopping" occurred because the Fifth Circuit was at the time considered more sympathetic to industry concerns than the D.C. Circuit.[29]

Although the ETS for benzene was blocked by the Fifth Circuit, OSHA proposed 1 ppm as a permanent PEL. Lengthy hearings were held in the summer of 1977. The proposal stimulated considerable opposition, particularly from corporate representatives and industry consultants. Five major objections were raised during the hearings:

- OSHA had not demonstrated excess leukemia risk among workers at the prevailing standard of 10 ppm.

- The lower standard was unnecessary because aplastic anemia could be a necessary precursor for leukemia, and a threshold above 10 ppm appeared to exist for aplastic anemia.[30]

• OSHA did not even attempt to quantify the number of cancers that might be prevented by the proposal.

• A quantitative risk assessment (QRA) performed by industrial consultant and Harvard physicist Richard Wilson showed that under certain assumptions the proposed standard would result in two fewer cancers every six years in a cohort of 30,000 exposed workers.[31]

• OSHA's feasibility analysis of the proposed rule did not contain a cost-benefit analysis (CBA) or cost-effectiveness analysis (CEA).[32]

Despite these criticisms, OSHA adopted the 1 ppm PEL as a permanent rule in February 1978. The agency's feasibility analysis estimated that the stricter standard would impose operating costs of $124 million in the first year and annual compliance costs of $74 million, in addition to initial capital investments of $267 million.[33] The agency nonetheless found that the stricter PEL would be "feasible" in the sense that the technology for compliance was available and compliance costs would not cripple or bankrupt the affected industries. The agency refused to adopt a standard lower than 1 ppm because of measurement difficulties and other feasibility considerations.[34]

The health justification for the new PEL was based on three premises: that benzene is a human carcinogen; that no safe levels of exposure have been demonstrated for carcinogens; and that the risk of contracting leukemia from exposure to benzene will decline as exposure levels are reduced. OSHA insisted that no further health justification was required by law. In fact, the agency rejected the need for a CBA and a QRA because it considered these tools unreliable and inconsistent with the agency's legislative mandate.

OSHA's reasoning was based in part on the generic carcinogen policy that was then in the proposal stage.[35] A key premise of the proposed policy was the no-threshold argument for carcinogens: namely, that any exposure, however small, to a carcinogenic chemical might pose some incremental risk of cancer. In light of that position, OSHA was proposing that all carcinogenic exposures be reduced to the lowest levels feasible. Thus the rationale offered for the final benzene standard was believed to be consistent with OSHA's proposed generic cancer policy.

To the Supreme Court

The final PEL for benzene of 1 ppm was also challenged by the API, again in the Fifth Circuit. The court unanimously struck down the 1 ppm rule, citing OSHA's failure to demonstrate a "reasonable relationship" between the costs of the new standard and the expected health benefits. Although it rejected a strict CBA test, the Fifth Circuit interpreted the "reasonably necessary or appropriate" language in section 3(8) of OSHA's statute as requiring a "reasonable relationship" between the costs of a standard and its benefits.[36]

The Fifth Circuit decision left OSHA dismayed, both because it blocked the benzene standard and because it seemed contrary to the agency's long-standing opposition to the use of CBAs in setting PELs for toxic chemicals. The Department of Justice agreed to represent OSHA in an appeal to the U.S. Supreme Court.

The Court accepted the appeal, creating expectations that a landmark opinion might be in the offing. On July 2, 1980—more than three years after OSHA had proposed the 1 ppm standard—the Supreme Court upheld the decision of the Fifth Circuit, thus blocking implementation of the 1 ppm standard.[37] The justices were so divided that a majority opinion could not be mustered. Although five justices concluded that OSHA's standard should be blocked, only four justices (a plurality) joined or concurred with the Court's opinion. In fact, the nine justices issued five separate opinions! The only opinion with four unqualified signatures was a blistering dissent written by Justice Thurgood Marshall. Even more confusing at the time was the plurality's decision not to resolve the cost-benefit question. Instead, they based their decision on OSHA's failure to show that benzene exposure creates a "significant" risk of cancer. One year later, however, in litigation on OSHA's cotton-dust standard, the Supreme Court finally resolved the cost-benefit issue in favor of OSHA.[38]

In the benzene and cotton-dust cases, the Supreme Court addressed four fundamental questions:

- Before regulating a chemical, must OSHA show that the chemical poses a "significant risk" to worker health? To do that, must OSHA do a formal risk assessment and quantify the expected health benefits?

- When OSHA issues a regulation, what kind of analysis must the agency make of the relationship between the potential health benefits of a rule and its economic costs? Is the use of CBA by OSHA required, permitted, or outlawed?

Table 4.1 The views of Supreme Court justices on key OSHA issues.

Justice	OSHA must show chemical poses "significant" risk	OSHA must show standard passes "benefit-cost" test	OSHA must adopt lowest feasible standard	Congress has unconstitutionally delegated power to OSHA
Blackman	No	No	Yes	No
Brennan	No	No	Yes	No
Marshall	No	No	Yes	No
White	No	No	Yes	No
Burger	Yes	No	No	Yes
Powell	Yes	Yes	?	?
Rehnquist	?[a]	No	No	Yes
Stewart	Yes	?	?	?
Stevens	Yes	No	Yes	No
Court vote	4–4–1	1–7–1	5–2–2	2–5–2
Status in law[b]	Yes	No	Yes	No

a. A question mark indicates that we have substantial doubts about a justice's view.
b. Current administrative law on the question.

• Once OSHA selects a chemical for regulation, must the agency choose the most protective standard that is "feasible"? What did Congress mean by "feasible"?

• Has Congress, by passing the Occupational Safety and Health Act without resolving key value trade-offs, delegated legislative authority to the executive branch in an unconstitutional manner?

Table 4.1 provides a summary of how each of the nine justices appeared to have resolved these questions. The "yes" or "no" assignments in the table are based on our reading of the opinions, concurrences, and dissents in the benzene and cotton-dust cases. In sum, it appears that the swing vote in these two cases was made by Justice Stevens, who wrote the plurality opinion in favor of QRA in the benzene case and then converted the dissenters in the benzene case into a majority against CBA in the cotton-dust case.

• OSHA's Second Benzene Rulemaking

The Supreme Court's benzene decision and the election of Ronald Reagan in November 1980 slowed but did not end pressure for a 1 ppm standard. On April 14, 1983, a consortium of labor unions and public-health groups petitioned OSHA administrator Thorne Auchter to issue an ETS for benzene. Auchter denied the ETS petition on July 1, 1983, but indicated that enough new data—especially positive animal studies—had accumulated to justify expedited consideration of a revised PEL.

Labor and Industry Negotiate

At the urging of OSHA, industry and labor groups began negotiations on the benzene standard in October 1983.[39] Labor participation included officials from the AFL-CIO, the United Steelworkers of America, the Oil, Chemical and Atomic Workers International, and the URW. Industry participation included officials from the Chemical Manufacturers Association, the Rubber Manufacturers Association, the American Iron and Steel Institute and the API. The meetings, organized by attorney Philip J. Harter, a negotiation expert, and Gerald W. Cormick of the Mediation Institute, were at times open to the press. The hope was that the parties could narrow their differences and possibly endorse a draft benzene standard to be proposed to OSHA. Yet the negotiations ended in March 1984 when the parties could not reach complete agreement on a proposal. It has been reported that there was agreement on many issues, but the ground rules for the exercise required that the parties agree to a comprehensive plan.

The real reasons for the failure to reach agreement are not obvious, and the stated reasons are complicated and in some cases conflicting. In our interviews with representatives of both sides, the following explanations were offered.

Although some industries were willing to accept a 1 ppm PEL, others—especially the steel industry—saw serious feasibility problems with that standard.

The resignation of OSHA head Thorne Auchter (who was enthusiastic about the negotiations), combined with the apathy and conflicting signals of OSHA staff members, caused each side to think it could do better without a negotiated standard.

The 1984 presidential election campaign and the campaign for presidency of the USW made it politically difficult for labor to take a cooperative posture.

Industry's insistence on a longer averaging period in the TWA (say, forty hours instead of eight hours) was perceived by some labor representatives as a bad precedent for future standards, especially by several labor leaders not directly involved in the benzene negotiations.

Industry's demand for a preamble finding no significant risk at 1 ppm (designed to protect firms from tort litigation) was unacceptable to labor because it might jeopardize the PEL on appeal to the courts.

New scientific data publicized during the negotiations—both more epidemiology and positive animal studies—caused labor to believe it could do better through normal rulemaking than through negotiations.

The nomination of Robert Rowland to run OSHA—a man deeply distrusted by labor (see Chapter 2)—caused labor representatives to be skeptical about a cooperative approach to benzene.[40] In any case, the negotiation experiment faltered, and labor took the issue to court.

Labor Goes to Court

On December 10, 1984, the United Steelworkers of America asked the D.C. Circuit Court of Appeals to compel OSHA to issue a new permanent benzene standard within eight months. The API and other corporate groups subsequently joined the suit as respondents.[41] At about this time the potential link between leukemia and occupational exposure to benzene received national publicity.

A scientific consultant to Shell Oil Company, Philip Cole, found an abnormally high rate of leukemias among workers at a Shell refinery where benzene was produced.[42] Eight workers employed at the refinery died of leukemia between 1973 and 1981, when only two leukemias would have been expected according to statistical averages. Cole believed that benzene exposure was "the most likely cause" of the excess leukemias. Unfortunately, precise data on the refinery workers' exposure to benzene are not available, so it is impossible to estimate a dose-response function.

The quality of the data on exposure is of critical importance to the policy debate. If the concentrations of benzene responsible for the excess leukemias were known to be close to the current PEL, then the case for tightening it would be very strong indeed. But if the workers had been exposed to extremely high concentrations (say, in excess of 100 ppm), then the benefits of reducing the PEL from 10 to 1 ppm could only be determined by guesswork and might actually be trivial or nonexistent.

Weeks after the publicity about leukemias at the Shell refinery, the *Wall Street Journal* printed an article based on an interview with NIOSH epidemiologist Robert Rinsky.[43] His new study purportedly showed a thirty-fold excess incidence of leukemia among workers exposed to benzene at 10 ppm. He also found an "appreciable" increased risk of leukemia among workers exposed to benzene at 1 ppm. Rinsky did not discuss his exact findings because the study was still under peer review. Apparently the study was based on a reconstruction of worker exposures in conjunction with the data from the earlier NIOSH study directed by Infante.

During the D.C. Circuit's period of deliberation, the API urged the new OSHA administrator, Robert Rowland, to propose a range of alternative PELS "because of the widely divergent interpretations of the available risk and feasibility evidence on benzene."[44] By opening a permanent rulemaking before the court decision, API argued, Rowland could "minimize the prospect of a short judicial timetable that might frustrate a full and evenhanded consideration of the issues." Rowland ultimately rejected the API's suggestion, approving instead a draft proposed standard of 1 ppm as an eight-hour TWA and 5 ppm as a ceiling limit averaged over a fifteen-minute period. The 1 ppm limit is identical to the limit Bingham had attempted to promulgate in 1978.

OSHA submitted the draft rule to the Office of Management and Budget (OMB) for review, as required under Executive Order 12291.[45] OMB, apparently dissatisfied with the proposal, extended its review well beyond the sixty-day period authorized in the executive order. Meanwhile, the leadership at OSHA was disrupted during the spring of 1985 following the resignation of Labor Secretary Ray Donovan and the appointment of William Brock to replace him. Then Rowland, whose appointment had never been approved by the Senate, resigned. After about six months of searching, Labor Secretary Brock nominated John Pendergrass to be the new head of OSHA in December 1985. Unlike his Reagan administration predecessors (Auchter and Rowland), Pendergrass was a career industrial hygienist with extensive corporate experience in health and safety issues. Shortly thereafter OSHA formally proposed a new PEL of 1 ppm for benzene, but it withdrew the short-term exposure limit of 5 ppm prior to publication, apparently because of objections by OMB. The 1 ppm standard was finalized by Pendergrass in the fall of 1987.

• EPA's Rulemaking on Benzene

The epidemiological evidence that benzene is a leukemogen, especially the 1976 NIOSH study by Infante, also caused EPA to consider

whether benzene should be a regulatory priority. On April 14, 1977—
several weeks before Bingham's announcement of the ETS at OSHA—
the Environmental Defense Fund (EDF) petitioned EPA to list benzene as a "hazardous air pollutant" pursuant to the agency's authority under section 112 of the Clean Air Act Amendments of 1970.
Section 112 defines a "hazardous air pollutant" as one that "may
cause, or contribute to, an increase in mortality or an increase in
serious irreversible, or incapacitating reversible, illness."[46]

Under the leadership of Douglas Costle, an attorney and a former
state environmental regulator, EPA decided to list benzene. The formal announcement estimated that as much as 260 million pounds of
benzene may be emitted into the air each year.[47] The principal sources
cited by EPA were chemical manufacturing facilities, petroleum refineries, gasoline storage and handling facilities, and automobiles.

For each pollutant listed under Section 112, uniform national emission standards are supposed to be set for all stationary sources at a
level that "protects the public health with an *ample margin of safety*"
(emphasis added).[48] Such standards must, according to the law, be
proposed within six months after the substance is listed, and final
standards must be issued within another six months. These provisions of section 112 presented EPA managers with severe logistical
and conceptual problems.

First, was it feasible to meet the six-month deadline? Agency procedure called for an assessment of benzene as a health risk prior to the
proposal of standards, with review by the public and the agency's
Science Advisory Board.[49] While some work on standards had been
done before the formal listing, much more needed to be done on the
extent of emissions from numerous sources and the feasibility of
emission-control technologies. Confessing this predicament, the
agency's listing notice stated that meeting the statutory deadline
"may not be feasible."[50]

More important, how was EPA to set emission standards for benzene that would protect the public health with an "ample margin of
safety"? The agency had several years earlier adopted a regulatory
policy which presumed that "some risk exists at any level of exposure
to carcinogenic chemicals."[51] Because of the disastrous economic implications of zero-emission standards for chemicals such as benzene,
EPA staff did not see how an ample margin of safety could realisti-
cally be assured. Instead, although it did not have statutory authorization to consider technology or economics, the agency announced
that its policy would be to reduce benzene emissions to the lowest

possible level, considering the availability of control technology and the relative risk to the public before and after the establishment of emission controls.[52]

The Carter administration's appointees to EPA, especially assistant administrator of air quality David Hawkins, who had been an attorney for NRDC, were clearly predisposed toward strict control of hazardous air pollutants. Yet progress toward adoption of benzene standards was extremely slow. In fact, it was not until April 1980 that the first standards were proposed for maleic anhydride plants.[53] When Carter lost to Reagan in 1980, the Carter appointees rushed to propose several more standards before the end of his term. In December 1980 and January 1981, standards were formally proposed for ethylbenzene and styrene plants, benzene storage vessels, and fugitive emission sources.[54] No proposals were issued regarding the other major sources of benzene emissions.

Environmentalists Pressure Gorsuch

The transition from the Carter to the Reagan administration and the appointment of Ann Gorsuch to replace Costle as head of EPA did not bring an immediate halt to preparation of final benzene standards. After analyzing public comments on the proposals and making some revisions, EPA staff in late May 1982 submitted a regulatory package to Kathleen Bennett, Hawkins's successor in the air quality office. In addition to the four final standards, the package contained a proposed standard for coke oven byproduct recovery plants.[55]

When nothing had happened after many months, environmentalists decided to try to use the statutory deadlines in Section 112 to their advantage. On December 23, 1982, EDF and NRDC notified Gorsuch of their intent to sue the agency for its inaction on benzene. Four months later the same groups notified the agency of their intent to sue about the lack of proposals for controlling benzene emissions from coke oven byproduct recovery plants and chemical manufacturing plants, and in gasoline marketing. In the spring of 1983, Ruckelshaus replaced Gorsuch at EPA; the benzene issue ultimately became the responsibility of Joseph Cannon, the next head of the air quality office.

Negotiations between EPA attorneys and environmentalists hit a snag when David Doniger of NRDC insisted on a written agreement that EPA would promulgate the benzene standards by September 1983.[56] In July, Democrat Mike Syner, the chairman of the House

Government Operations Subcommittee on Environment, Energy, and Natural Resources, held oversight hearings on why EPA had not set standards to protect the public from exposure to benzene emissions in gasoline vapors at service stations. On the day of the hearings, NRDC and EDF filed suit in the U.S. district court for the District of Columbia seeking to force EPA to set final standards for benzene emissions.[57]

The explicit statutory deadlines combined with the EDF/NRDC lawsuit forced EPA to make decisions, but there was no consensus inside the agency about what to do. The air quality and policy offices were in an overt and heated dispute.[58] The key policy analysts were arguing that revised emission and risk estimates demonstrated that ambient benzene exposures did not constitute a significant risk. Moreover, they argued that the standards would not be very cost effective. In contrast, the air quality office professionals from Research Triangle Park, North Carolina—who had developed the standards—saw no compelling rationale to retreat on the proposals. The issue ultimately went to Cannon and then to Ruckelshaus for resolution.

In December 1983, before the court proceedings were resolved, Ruckelshaus approved Cannon's recommendation. The earlier proposals to regulate maleic anhydride plants, ethylbenzene/styrene plants, and benzene storage vessels were withdrawn on the basis that these sources presented "insignificant" risks.[59] A final rule was issued covering fugitive emissions, and a new rule was proposed covering coke oven byproduct recovery plants. The two rules to be adopted, EPA analysts said, would control more than 70 percent of the stationary sources of benzene emissions.[60] These proposals were published in the *Federal Register* in the spring of 1984. In the interim the D.C. district court ordered EPA to resolve the fate of the benzene rules by May 23, 1984.[61] After receiving public comments, EPA published the two actions in final form with little revision in June 1984.[62]

EPA's Reasoning

EPA defended its final benzene decisions primarily on the basis of risk estimates produced by the agency's Carcinogen Assessment Group. The estimates, summarized in Table 4.2, are based on exposure estimates from atmospheric dispersion models, relative risks from occupational epidemiological studies, and a no-threshold model that assumes leukemia incidence is linearly related to benzene exposure, even at very low levels of exposure. EPA insisted that the linear,

Table 4.2 EPA's risk estimates for benzene: baseline impacts for stationary sources.

Emission source category	Number of affected plants	Maximum lifetime risk	Cases of excess leukemia per year
Fugitive emissions	128	1.5×10^{-3}	0.45
Maleic anhydride	7	7.6×10^{-5}	0.029
Ethylbenzene/ styrene	13	1.4×10^{-5}	0.0057
Benzene storage	126	3.6×10^{-4}	0.043
Coke byproduct plants	42	6.4×10^{-3}	2.2

Source: Federal Register, 49 (1984): 23492, 23525.

no-threshold model is conservative (that is, it tends to provide an "upper bound" on true risk) and that it has "the best, albeit limited, scientific basis of any current mathematical extrapolation model."[63] The standards adopted for fugitive sources and coke byproduct plants did not require zero emissions. Instead, EPA's definition of the "best available technology" (BAT) mandated the lowest emissions achievable. In defending its withdrawal of the three other standards, EPA pointed to the guideline of an excess 1 in 1,000 lifetime risk to represent "significance," as espoused by Justice Stevens in the OSHA benzene case. Although OSHA and EPA are governed by different laws, EPA lawyers believed that the Supreme Court's significance doctrine was applicable to the laws of both agencies.

The decision by Ruckelshaus was criticized by interest groups on both sides. Representatives of industry argued that benzene should never have been listed as a hazardous air pollutant in the first place. According to these critics, the excess incidence of leukemia observed among workers heavily exposed to benzene is unlikely to arise from ambient exposures, which are often three orders of magnitude smaller than the occupational exposures. At such low concentrations, it is argued that a threshold for carcinogenicity is likely, especially because there are no data demonstrating that benzene reacts chemically with DNA and because it is suspected that the threshold for benzene's toxic effects on the blood is relatively high (10 to 35 ppm).

The NRDC, on the other hand, criticized the agency for withdrawing the three standards, suggesting that the risk estimates were unreliable and were also a legally impermissible basis for withdrawal. In a lawsuit contesting the withdrawal decisions, NRDC argued that

EPA did not have the authority to avoid taking responsibility for standard setting on the grounds of insignificant risk. Standards must be set at the level that "protects the public health with an ample margin of safety," a mandate that leaves no room for significance judgments. In addition, NRDC charged that EPA ignored more recent animal and human studies that would have generated higher risk estimates than those reported in Table 4.2. At this writing the NRDC lawsuit has not yet been decided.

■ Alternative Approaches to Standard Setting

During the Carter and Reagan years, the benzene controversy became a forum for debate about how strictly federal agencies should regulate human exposures to toxic chemicals. On the surface the debate appeared to be a narrow legal dispute about the definition of such words as "significant," "feasible," "safe," and "reasonable." But as all the participants understood, the real debate was about conflicting values and interests. The key legislative phrases were not self-defining, and alternative interpretations were influenced by the interests of the parties and their beliefs about what constitutes appropriate social policy on suspected carcinogens.

On one extreme is the view that standards should protect each citizen's absolute right to health. At the other extreme is the view that health risks are dealt with optimally by markets and that there is no justification for standard setting by federal agencies. Between these extremes are several approaches to standard setting that place varying degrees of emphasis on health, technological, and economic considerations. This section describes the various decision rules that were prominent in the policy debates about benzene, including the problems associated with each. The key concepts are lowest feasible risk, elimination of significant risk, and balancing of costs and benefits.

Lowest Feasible Risk

Proponents of feasibility analysis argue that human exposure to benzene and other carcinogens should be reduced to the lowest feasible levels. The position was stated succinctly by Ruth Ruttenberg and Eula Bingham in the OSHA context: "Our overall goal should be workplaces free of carcinogenic risk. While issues of feasibility may sometimes prevent such risk-free environments, we should not lose sight of the goal, and we should continue to work towards it whenever possible."[64] This formulation of OSHA's mission was the intellectual basis of the agency's final 1978 benzene rule and its proposed generic carcinogen policy.

The lowest-feasible-risk position asserts that health protection is the preeminent value in OSHA and EPA decisions. Each worker has a right to safe and healthy working conditions, and each citizen has a right not to be victimized by hazardous air pollution. Stated negatively, it is not fair or equitable for workers or citizens to be subjected to carcinogenic risks, even if they or others will reap benefits from the situation creating the risks. In philosophical terms the position is incompatible with the utilitarian assumptions of cost-benefit analysis. Feasibility is not viewed as a competing right or value, but rather as pragmatic constraint on the achievement of what is right and proper. Supporters of this view point to section 6(b)(5) of the OSHA statute, where Congress directs OSHA to set standards such that "no employee will suffer material impairment of health or functional capacity even if such employee has regular exposure to the hazard dealt with by such standard for the period of his working life." This language stresses the individualized nature of the worker's right to health protection.

Justice Brennan expressed for the Supreme Court the view that Congress intended OSHA to conduct a very special kind of feasibility analysis: "Congress itself defined the basic relationship between costs and benefits, by placing the 'benefits' of worker health above all other considerations save those making attainment of the 'benefit' unachievable."[65] The health-maximizing focus of this sort of feasibility analysis does seem to be related to certain professional orientations and habits of mind. Proponents of this view frequently are in the health-related professions (safety engineering, industrial hygiene, toxicology, environmental health, and public health), although there are important differences among these professional subcultures. For example, the National Safety Council's manual for safety engineers speaks of industrial accidents and the "needless destruction of life and limb" as "moral evil." Treating workers' health as a special kind of good underlies the institutional vitality of an agency such as OSHA.[66] Agreement on a simple moral principle such as health protection can help an organization sustain morale and recruit likeminded and effective employees.[67]

The lowest-feasible-risk doctrine also arises from broader beliefs about the relative powers of employers and workers in the marketplace and in politics. Those who believe that the interests of workers in healthy and safe work environments tend to be underrepresented in collective bargaining and politics have a strong reason to support an activist, nonbalancing interpretation of OSHA's statute. According to this view, OSHA should be a partisan advocate for the health interests of workers, just as contrary views and interests have their advocates in society. The decision of Congress to make OSHA a part of the Department of Labor (instead of an independent commission) lends credence to this inherently partisan conception of OSHA's mission.

The same principle is often advanced to justify nonbalancing approaches to environmental control. If polluting industries are politically powerful and environmental groups are relatively impotent, then it is appropriate for EPA to take a pro-environment position in standard setting. That, it is argued, is the nature of democratic pluralism.

Advocates of workers' rights and environmental protection often recognize the need for OSHA or EPA to consider feasibility. Unfortunately, the operational meaning of this word for the practice of standard setting is not obvious. One view is that there is no real lowest-feasible-risk standard; there are only successively more stringent and expensive limits on emissions or exposures.[68] What is feasible in the future is itself a function of how much manpower and resources are devoted to research and development. The concept of technical feasibility might come down to the amount of resources invested to modify existing production processes or invent and deploy new ones. At some point, a judgment that a standard is not feasible may embody implicit assumptions about the incremental benefits and costs of more stringent limitations on chemical exposure. Regardless of how stringent the standards are made, one might argue that the underlying value trade-offs should be made explicit, so that workers, businesses, and the general citizenry can participate in the process.

Proponents of feasibility analysis believe otherwise. Their view is that a standard's feasibility can be judged by whether compliance technologies are available and are affordable by the affected industries. Justice Brennan expressed this view for the Court majority in the cotton-dust case: "Congress was concerned that the Act might be thought to require achievement of absolute safety, an impossible standard, and therefore insisted that health and safety goals be capable of economic and technological accomplishment."[69] A body of principles and case law has emerged to clarify the meaning of feasibility analysis.

A standard may be considered technologically feasible even if no existing devices would allow industry to comply with the standard. In litigation on OSHA's vinyl chloride rule, a federal court emphasized the "technology-forcing" nature of the agency's authority: "[OSHA] may raise standards which require improvements in existing technologies or which require the development of new technology, and [OSHA] is not limited to issuing standards based solely on devices already fully developed."[70] One court noted that OSHA can require industries to meet chemical exposure limits never achieved anywhere "so long as it presents substantial evidence that companies acting vigorously and in good faith can develop the technology."[71] Indeed, OSHA may impose extremely stringent limits on chemical exposure if it "gives industry a reasonable amount of time to develop new technology."

There remains more doubt about the correct interpretation of "economic feasibility." It is clear that federal agencies will estimate the economic costs of proposed standards and determine whether or not the standards are "affordable" by affected industries. In reviewing OSHA's expensive regulation of coke oven emissions, a federal court said that "Congress did not intend to eliminate all health hazards to industrial employees at the price of crippling an industry or rendering it extinct."[72] The same court emphasized, though, that an expensive PEL is not necessarily economically infeasible: "Although we are very sensitive to the financial implications of the standard and have endeavored to carefully weigh its effects upon the well-being of the industry, we are not persuaded that its implementation would precipitate anything approaching the 'massive dislocation' which would characterize an economically infeasible standard."

Although some troubled firms may find regulatory standards particularly expensive or even financially prohibitive, courts have not excused individual firms from health standards. On the contrary, one court insisted: "It would appear to be consistent with the purposes of the Act to envisage the economic demise of an employer who has lagged behind the industry in protecting the health and safety of employees and is consequently financially unable to comply with new standards as quickly as other employers."[73]

In summary, the feasibility approach calls for the lowest exposures to carcinogenic chemicals that are within the technological and financial capabilities of regulated industries.[74] On this view, suggestions that the marginal health benefits of standards should somehow be weighed against their marginal economic costs are to be rejected on both technical and philosophical grounds. Cost-benefit comparisons are viewed as both unreliable and immoral components of standard setting.

Elimination of Significant Risk

A second approach to standard setting, which arose in the OSHA context and was later used at EPA, is the significant-risk doctrine. It asserts that federal agencies should concentrate on eliminating "significant" carcinogenic risks. Justice Stevens expressed this view in the Court's plurality opinion in the benzene case. In rejecting OSHA's rationale for the 1 ppm PEL for benzene, that opinion states: "We think it is clear that the statute was not designed to require employers to provide absolutely risk-free workplaces whenever it is technologically feasible to do so, so long as the cost is not great enough to destroy an entire industry. Rather, both the language and structure of the Act, as well as its legislative history, indicate that it was intended to require the elimination, as far as feasible, of significant risks of harm."[75] Note that the first sentence of this passage specifically rejects the lowest-feasible-risk doctrine. Instead, exposure to a carcinogen has to be shown to pose a *significant* risk. Then the level of exposure should be lowered to reduce the risk to insignificance or, if that is impossible, to the lowest feasible level. The plurality expressed no opinion about whether benzene exposures at 10 ppm do, in fact, constitute a significant risk. The issue was simply remanded to OSHA for further consideration because the agency had made no attempt to show that benzene exposure carried a significant risk of harm.

As a matter of law, the Stevens opinion is only a partial confirmation of the Fifth Circuit's opinion. Without endorsing cost-benefit analysis, the plurality confirmed the Fifth Circuit's view that section 3(8) of the act places some additional limitation on OSHA's authority to regulate chemicals, beyond the feasibility language contained in section 6(b)(5). In order to show that a 1 ppm PEL for benzene is "reasonably necessary and appropriate to provide safe or healthful employment," OSHA must find that benzene exposures at 10 ppm pose a significant risk to health and that exposures of 1 ppm will significantly reduce the risk.

The significant-risk doctrine rejects zero risk as the goal of OSHA's rulemaking. Justice Stevens insisted that "safe" is not the same as "risk-free," pointing to a variety of risks in daily life that Americans find acceptable. He offered "driving a car or even breathing city air" as examples of risky activities in daily life, yet he believed few people would consider these activities "unsafe." Thus OSHA standards ought to aim at an acceptable risk, not zero risk, of cancer.

The significant-risk doctrine is based partly on economic concerns. For carcinogens, OSHA under Bingham had argued that the statute required exposure levels to be set at zero or, if that is impossible, at the lowest feasible levels. The Court plurality rejected that view: "In the absence of a clear mandate in the Act, it is unreasonable to assume that Congress intended to give the Secretary the unprecedented power over American industry that would result from the Government's view of sections 3(8) and 6(b)(5), coupled with OSHA's cancer policy . . . The Government's theory would give OSHA power to impose enormous costs that might produce little, if any, discernible benefit." Chief Justice Burger highlighted this point in his concurring opinion, arguing that OSHA does not have the power to squander national resources in an attempt to eliminate *de minimis* risks.[76] Thus, the significant-risk doctrine provides some economic protection for firms whose workers are exposed to insignificant risks.

The significant-risk notion is not simply a constraint on the stringency of OSHA standards; it is also a suggestion that rulemaking priorities be directed toward the most important chemical risks. OSHA has extremely limited rulemaking resources.[77] Even if the budget could somehow be increased, there are probably political limits on the regulatory costs that can be imposed on the private sector.

Under these conditions the agency cannot regulate all risky chemicals. The choices of which chemicals to regulate and when to regulate them are critical public-health matters. If OSHA's priority-setting process were indisputedly rational, there would be less justification for a significant-risk doctrine. Although OSHA's generic carcinogen rule does not forbid the use of analytical methods in setting priorities, the history of OSHA regulation suggests that priorities are likely to be set in an ad hoc and idiosyncratic manner. Most chemicals are regulated in response to petitions from labor unions or public-health groups, with little analysis by the agency of alternative regulatory targets. Moreover, courts are reluctant to review directly the internal priorities of regulatory agencies.[78] By requiring OSHA to show significant risk as a prelude to standard setting, the plurality was insisting on some analysis in priority setting.

The plurality urged that "the risk from a toxic substance be quantified sufficiently to enable the Secretary to characterize it as significant in an understandable way." Chief Justice Burger conceded that "it is difficult to say precisely what this means," but the plurality opinion emphasized the scientific elements of the significant-risk determination. The "finding" of significant risk must be "supported by a reputable body of scientific thought." The plurality argued that industry must be allowed to offer "expert testimony" or "empirical evidence" that a particular risk is "insignificant." At one point the plurality described the threshold finding of significant risk as "not unlike the threshold finding that a chemical is toxic or a physical agent is harmful."

The phrase "significant risk" appears nowhere in the plain language of the act or in the relevant legislative history. The Stevens opinion conceded this point but argued that the concept of significant risk was implied by the act and its history. Justice Marshall and the dissenters saw no such implication, describing the significant-risk doctrine as "a fabrication bearing no connection with the acts or intentions of Congress." Later Marshall called the new doctrine "the plurality's own invention" and said "it can be understood only as reflecting the personal views of the plurality as to the proper allocation of resources for safety in the American workplace."

The significant-risk doctrine was originally espoused by only four justices, and therefore, its legal importance was in doubt in 1980.[79] Soon after the Court's benzene decision, Judge Skelly Wright of the D.C. Circuit speculated that there was actually a five-person majority on the Court "for the view that section 3(8) does not place on OSHA any threshold burden of proving 'significant harm.' "[80] In the cotton-dust case, however, a majority of the Court (the four dissenters in the benzene case plus Stevens) upheld OSHA's standard while delivering an opinion that "all section 6(b)(5) standards must be addressed to 'significant risks' of material health impairment."[81]

OSHA, EPA, and the federal courts have taken the new doctrine seriously. In the cotton-dust case the Supreme Court was satisfied with OSHA's evidence that exposure to cotton dust creates a significant risk of byssinosis (brown-lung disease). In litigation on OSHA's lead standard, the D.C. Circuit decided that "OSHA has clearly met the section 3(8) threshold test of proving 'significant harm' described by the American Petroleum Institute plurality."[82] The Fifth Circuit struck down OSHA's cotton gin regulations on grounds of "insignificant risk."[83] OSHA itself took specific action to incorporate the new doctrine into an amended version of the generic carcinogen rule.[84] And we observed earlier that EPA used the doctrine in 1984 to support its withdrawal of several benzene standards under section 112 of the Clean Air Act Amendments of 1970.

It is difficult to predict how the significant-risk concept will be defined and applied in future cases, but there are some hints in Justice Stevens's opinion. He described an extra lifetime mortality risk of 1 in 1,000 as something that "a reasonable person might well consider significant and take appropriate steps to decrease or eliminate it."[85] OSHA has used this numerical guideline to support recent proposals aimed at cutting worker exposures to arsenic and asbestos.[86] EPA has used it to support some benzene standards and to withdraw others.

The Stevens opinion also defined significance in a comparative context, stating that it is possible to make "a rational judgment about the *relative* significance of risks associated with exposure to a particular carcinogen" (emphasis added).[87] That passage can be interpreted as authorization for OSHA to employ "comparative risk assessment," a technique advocated by Professor Richard Wilson and Republican Congressman Don Ritter that uses QRA to determine acceptable risk.[88] For example, the carcinogenic risk associated with workers' exposure to an industrial chemical might be judged acceptable if it is equal to or less than the normal industrial accident risk faced by blue-collar workers. Harvey Brooks has suggested that normal accident risks could be assigned a safety factor, which could serve as the quantitative threshold of acceptable risk.[89]

OSHA's justification for the final arsenic standard is of special interest because it contains the agency's first published analysis of the significant-risk question. Five factors entered into OSHA's determination that arsenic posed a significant risk: the quality of the data, the reasonableness of assumptions underlying the agency's QRA, the statistical significance of the agency's findings, the severity of the harm presented, and the numerical significance of the arsenic risk relative to other occupational risk factors.[90]

The health risks of exposure to arsenic, ethylene dibromide, ethylene oxide, and asbestos were deemed significant in subsequent OSHA rulemakings. Table 4.3 summarizes quantitative estimates of selected occupational health risks as published in these rulemakings. The cancer risks of occupational exposure to radiation and other occupational accident risks are presented for comparison. In the case of benzene, the studies submitted to the OSHA docket projected

Table 4.3 Quantitative estimates of selected occupational accident and health risks.

Chemical or occupation	Exposure assumption	Condition	Excess lifetime incidence per 1,000 workers
Arsenic	500 μg/m^3	Lung cancer	148–425
EDB	20 ppm	Cancer	70–110
Ethylene oxide	50 ppm	Cancer	63–109
Benzene	10 ppm	Leukemia	14–152
Asbestos	2 fibers/cm	Asbestosis, lung cancer	44–56
Fire fighting	—	Sudden death	27
Radiation	5 rems	Cancer	17–29
Mining and quarrying	—	Sudden death	20
All manufacturing jobs	—	Sudden death	2.7
All service jobs	—	Sudden death	1.6

Source: Occupational Safety and Health Administration, "Occupational Exposure to Benzene," *Federal Register,* 50 (1985): 50538–50539.

lifetime risks of 14 to 207 deaths per 1,000 workers at 10 ppm,[91] although Wilson's original estimate in 1977 was slightly less than one excess death per 1,000 workers. The range of risk for benzene that OSHA now projects is 44 to 152 deaths per 1,000 workers, even though Justice Stevens seemed to be impressed with Wilson's earlier estimate.[92] In Chapter 6 we take a careful look at the assumptions and controversies that surround these risk estimates.

OSHA's use of comparative risk assessment to show significance is likely to produce heated controversy. The key value judgment is that current accident risks are acceptable and that OSHA's mission is to regulate only those risks that are above this acceptable level. Wilson has used such an approach to argue that the risk of leukemia from exposure to 10 ppm of benzene is not serious enough to warrant tighter regulation.[93] But according to other views of significance, comparative risk assessment is unacceptable. If OSHA was created because Congress regarded the average level of industrial accident risk as too high, then it makes little sense to use industrial accidents as a guideline for acceptable health risk.[94] As a matter of fact, Congress may have intended more stringent protection against chronic health risks than against accident risks. That would help explain why section 6(b)(5) of the OSHA statute was adopted and applied exclusively to toxic materials and harmful physical agents. One can also argue that chemical risks are of greater social significance than industrial accident risks because workers do not know about insidious contaminants and because the public has special fears about cancer as a painful way to die. Moreover, people may perceive carcinogenic risks as less voluntary or controllable than accident risks. Indeed, some health advocates reject a comparative approach per se because they believe that any incremental risk of cancer, however small, is unacceptable and ethically significant.

The significant-risk doctrine places a somewhat higher analytical burden on those who wish to regulate a potential carcinogen than does the lowest-feasible-risk notion. Not all suspected carcinogens are treated equally; only those chemicals shown to pose a significant risk of cancer will be regulated, focusing limited administrative resources on the most important health risks. In addition, the significant-risk doctrine places a constraint on the stringency of standards. If exposure to a carcinogen is reduced to the point that the residual cancer risk is insignificant, then no further tightening of the standard is appropriate.

Balancing Costs and Health Benefits

In contrast to the views that feasibility or significant risk provides an appropriate basis for standard setting is the view that a rational public policy toward carcinogens must balance explicitly the benefits of risk reduction against the costs. OSHA has historically rejected this approach, arguing that the most protective PEL should be selected for carcinogens without regard to the relative health benefits and costs. As noted earlier, OSHA has defined feasibility solely in terms of technology and industry affordability, with no direct balancing of the incremental costs and benefits of alternative PELs. EPA has, at least until recently, also resisted this approach when setting standards for airborne carcinogens. The positions of these federal agencies have stimulated intense opposition from both business leaders and professional economists, who are the primary proponents of the balancing approach.

Balancers dispute the notion that workers have rights to risk-free jobs. They argue that many workers take and retain hazardous jobs in exchange for wage premiums and other benefits, so workers themselves do not appear to regard health protection as an absolute value.[95] The balancing approach would have OSHA treat health as a fungible good just as workers do. In fact, it is argued, making jobs risk-free could be detrimental to all concerned because workers would lose wage premiums, and firms and consumers would incur the potentially enormous costs of making jobs free of risk. Harvard economist Richard Zeckhauser has made this point to OSHA: "In many areas [of life] we tolerate positive, often substantial, levels of risk, despite the availability of technologies to reduce them. We have decided, at least implicitly, that the costs of further reducing these risks outweigh the benefits. The OSHA concept of feasibility denies the legitimacy of such choices."[96]

The balancing approach does not assume that the operation of real-world labor markets necessarily results in optimal levels of exposure to chemical carcinogens. Markets suffer from a variety of defects, such as imperfect worker information and imbalance in the bargaining relationships of employees and employers. The mission of OSHA should be, according to the balancing approach, to devise standards that approximate the outcomes of perfectly functioning labor markets.[97]

To illustrate the utilitarian nature of the balancing approach, it is useful to consider a hypothetical example. Suppose a reduction in the PEL for benzene from 10 to 1 ppm will (with certainty) avert three cases of fatal cancer per year in a stable population of 30,000 exposed workers. If the stricter PEL is adopted, assume that consumers of benzene-related products will (with certainty) pay extra costs of $3 million per year.

A balancer would endorse the lower PEL if and only if each member of society is willing to pay at least $100 per year to eliminate the excess annual cancer risk of one in 10,000. This figure is found by adding up what workers and other citizens are willing to pay for the lower PEL (altruistic payments do count as "benefits" of the lower PEL). If society as a whole is willing to pay at least $3 million for the lower PEL, then it is theoretically possible to compensate citizens for the extra costs of the lower PEL (assuming zero transaction costs). A proposal that passes this theoretical compensation test is called a "potential Pareto improvement" by economists. It is in this sense that economists say the lower PEL should be adopted only if "benefits outweigh costs."

The phrase "cost-benefit analysis," which has a precise meaning to professional economists, is often used in a more general way by business leaders. Their notion is that an agency should consider both the costs and benefits of proposed standards and make a judgment about the proper balance. Sometimes business leaders have in mind what economists call cost-effectiveness analysis (CEA). Under this approach, the incremental cost per case of cancer avoided is calculated for alternative standards at various plants. An attempt is made to equalize the marginal cost of cancer prevention among plants and standards, although the maximum expenditure that is appropriate to prevent a statistical case of cancer is left as a political judgment for regulators. In any case, both CBA and CEA call for some balancing of economic costs and health benefits.

The balancer does not insist that losers actually be compensated after the lower PEL is adopted. Nor does the balancer consider the distribution of benefits and costs or the characteristics of the "winners" and "losers" resulting from the lower PEL. Critics of balancing, such as Nicholas Ashford, object that this approach ignores distributional issues: "The most serious limitation [of cost-benefit analysis], however, lies in the failure to successfully deal with the fact that the cost and benefit streams accrue to different parties. One person's benefit cannot be neatly traded off from another's cost."[98] This objection has special appeal to health advocates because, under the CBA approach, one worker's or citizen's health may be compromised for another person's economic benefit.

Balancers do not find this objection persuasive for a variety of reasons. Health benefits are not viewed as different from other kinds of benefits. Instead, all benefits and costs are assumed to be fungible, because they all contribute to individual happiness—which utilitarians argue is the ultimate moral test.

On the distributional question, many balancers are prepared to assume that on average the distribution of happiness in the society will not be made less equitable by the cost-benefit approach. They argue further that the potential beneficiaries of OSHA or EPA regulations are not necessarily economically disadvantaged citizens who are especially worthy of governmental protection. Steel, oil, chemical, and atomic workers are well paid by most standards, in part because of the nature of their jobs and in part because of the strength of their unions.[99] The major beneficiaries of air pollution control are often middle-class citizens. Nor are the costs of OSHA or EPA standards borne primarily by stockholders, corporate executives, and affluent people. Whenever standards reduce corporate profits, taxpayers suffer because the government loses revenue from corporate income taxes. Workers may well pay the costs in reduced wages, and consumers pay the costs in higher prices and reduced consumption. Thus Zeckhauser, for example, argues that all segments of society ultimately bear the costs of occupational health standards.

Even if some poor citizens are made worse off by a particular policy that relies on CBA, the balancers take a long-run view. Any losses will tend to be offset by gains over time, and ultimately most citizens—even most poor citizens—should be made better off by the CBA approach. If it could somehow be demonstrated that identifiable groups of citizens were consistently harmed by the balancing approach, a case could be made for a lump-sum transfer of resources to these persons. Balancers would, for the sake of efficiency, make this transfer through income-security policy, not regulatory policy.

The balancing approach is analytically even more demanding than the significant-risk doctrine because it requires much more information: quantitative risk estimates and cost estimates for each regulatory alternative and good estimates of society's willingness to pay for reductions in the cancer rate. Implementation of the balancing approach would clearly require that OSHA and EPA be transformed from advocacy agencies into analytical shops that work to advance social welfare, broadly defined.

Advocates of CBA suffered a major setback when the Supreme Court upheld OSHA's cotton-dust standard. Justice Brennan's opinion for the five-member majority stated that "cost-benefit analysis is not required by the statute because feasibility analysis is."[100] The passages in his opinion appear to constitute a *de jure* prohibition on the use of CBA by OSHA in setting PELs for toxic chemicals.

The role for CBA in OSHA decision making has not, however, been obliterated by Brennan's opinion. The Court did not preclude the use of CBA in selecting regulatory priorities.[101]

In addition, Congress has considered legislation that would impose cost-benefit tests on the rulemaking activities of all federal regulatory agencies, including OSHA.[102] In actual practice, OSHA and EPA under Reagan have conducted CBAs despite the legal issues. OMB actually requires that OSHA and EPA make such analyses prior to promulgating rules, even though it may not be lawful for these agencies to weaken a standard because of cost-benefit considerations.[103]

• Implications of the Alternative Approaches

What are the practical consequences of conducting rulemakings according to these various decision rules? In particular, how might they effect the process and outcomes of standard setting? Although it is not possible to answer these questions without a larger empirical inquiry, in this section we use the benzene controversy to generate some predictions and hypotheses.

The Role for Risk Quantification

If decision rules call for reducing emissions or exposures to the lowest feasible levels, then quantitative risk assessments—even if possible—are unnecessary. In the case of benzene, OSHA would only have to answer the question, "Does human exposure to benzene at 10 ppm create an incremental risk of leukemia?" If the answer is yes, then exposures must be reduced to the level necessary to eliminate the extra risk of leukemia. If such a level is zero (assuming no threshold) or impossible to achieve, then exposures must be reduced to the lowest levels compatible with technological feasibility and economic affordability. Since quantitative estimates of carcinogenic risk are not required, wrangling over the reliability of quantification is unnecessary and unproductive.

If, on the other hand, federal agencies are to regulate only significant risks, then a merely qualitative risk assessment may not be sufficient. The Supreme Court's plurality opinion in the benzene case expressed a clear preference for significant-risk judgments based on quantitative risk assessments. Even so, it is not clear that quantification is always required. Justice Stevens said that the doctrine is not intended to be a "mathematical straitjacket," and Justice Powell's concurring opinion stressed that "OSHA's hands" are not "tied when reasonable quantification cannot be accomplished by known methods." Powell believes that significance can sometimes be demonstrated by "the weight of expert testimony and opinion," even without quantification.[104]

In contrast, cost-benefit balancing by its very nature demands quantification. The number of cancers to be prevented by lowering the PEL for benzene from 10 to 1 ppm must be estimated in order to weigh the marginal costs of the tighter PEL against the marginal benefits. Advocates of CBA insist that some type of quantification is always possible, even if the estimates must be subjective, with huge amounts of uncertainty. Techniques are available to incorporate uncertainty into CBA. Scientific ignorance, they argue, is not a decisive obstacle to standard setting based on CBA.[105]

The Role of Cost Information

Alternative decision rules also influence the type of economic analysis that an agency will perform. The lowest-feasible-risk rule and the significant-risk rule both require federal agencies to determine the financial capabilities of affected industries, as well as the costs to firms of selected standards. In contrast, the CBA approach requires that more attention be given to the incremental cost of various control levels and less attention to affordability.

Determining financial feasibility (that is, what additional costs an industry can bear without having to close a number of plants) is a complex business. Factors that are likely to be important include projected industry profit margins, changes in demand for the industry's products when prices change, the rate of growth of the market, the debt burdens faced by major firms, and projected production capacities and costs of major foreign competitors. If an industry appears "healthy" on these dimensions, then a tighter standard—even if extremely costly—may pose no risk of harming or destroying the industry. In contrast, an industry that is in extremely poor financial condition might not be able to survive tighter standards even if those standards entail relatively modest capital and operating costs.

In contrast, classic CBA is not concerned with the financial condition of firms and industries. A standard that maximizes net benefits is favored even if the affected industry is financially troubled and likely to collapse. Alternatively, a stricter standard with negative net benefits would be rejected, even if the industry could easily afford the costs. Instead of weighing compliance costs against the financial health of the industry, the strict academic version of cost-benefit doctrine calls for comparing the marginal compliance costs to the marginal gains (in willingness to pay for health) of progressively tighter standards.

The distinction between economic feasibility analysis and CBA is not always appreciated, despite the profound implications for regulatory policy. Firms in an industry with "deep pockets" are much more likely to have to meet very strict standards under the feasibility rule than under strict CBA.

Health Consequences of Alternative Decision Rules

A common assertion in debates about regulatory policy is that feasibility analysis will be more protective of health than cost-benefit balancing. When we consider the interaction between priority setting and standard setting, this assertion is not necessarily so self-evident.

Concede for the moment that a carcinogenic chemical will be regulated more strictly under feasibility considerations than under cost-benefit considerations (although this assumption may be erroneous in cases where an industry is financially troubled). John Mendeloff has argued that there is a trade-off between the strictness of a regulation and what he calls its "extensiveness" (the total number of toxic chemicals regulated). Under this theory, OSHA will regulate fewer chemicals if it is forced to mandate the lowest feasible exposures for each chemical targeted for regulation. Mendeloff concludes: "Viewed in this perspective, the Supreme Court's recent cotton dust decision, which restricts the use of cost-benefit analysis in favor of more protective criteria for standard-setting, might actually end up diminishing OSHA's contribution to worker health."[106]

In support of Mendeloff's position, one can say that an industry's opposition to a proposed standard probably increases with the strictness of the standard. As industry opposition becomes more intense, a regulatory agency's staff must respond to larger numbers of docket submissions, pressure from OMB economists, adversarial reports from industry consultants, and intricate lawsuits. The monetary, legal, and political resources of the agency are spread thin, reducing the resources available to regulate other toxic chemicals. W. Kip Viscusi argues that industrial backlash was especially damaging during Bingham's years at OSHA: "The moratorium on new health risk regulations during the final three years of the Carter Administration can be traced to the uncertainties raised by the benzene case and related court tests of OSHA's authority. Challenges to OSHA's interpretation of its legislative mandate in effect brought the regulatory rulemaking process to a standstill. The agency's myopic commitment to an absolute interpretation of its authority may have jeopardized the lives of thousands of workers who could have been protected if OSHA had regulated health risks in a more balanced manner."[107] According to this view, a balancing approach to standard setting at OSHA would have done more for worker health than feasibility analysis.

The Viscusi critique is misplaced if OSHA is viewed as a prisoner of its legislative mandate. Perhaps Bingham and her predecessors had no lawful choice other than to adopt the lowest-feasible-level interpretation. Yet OSHA could have taken the initiative to recommend legislative change, as Ruckelshaus did (unsuccessfully) for many of EPA's authorizing statutes.[108] Moreover, courts often give agencies some leeway in interpreting vague statutory demands, so OSHA could have advocated a legal position more permissive of cost-benefit considerations. Litigation might have proceeded differently if the courts had been asked to impose upon OSHA a stricter statutory interpretation than the agency preferred. A test case of this hypothesis will be judicial review of EPA's legal position on standards for hazardous air pollutants under section 112 of the Clean Air Act. The agency has abandoned a zero-risk interpretation of the law and is trying in various ways to consider costs and benefits.

• Conclusion

What are we to make of the various decision rules that have been proposed to guide standard setting by federal agencies? Documents such as rulemaking rationales in the *Federal Register*, opinions of federal judges, and briefs of litigants imply that there *are* semantically correct ways to define key words such as "significant," "feasible," "ample margin of safety," and "reasonably necessary." We contend that although the English language is not infinitely elastic, there is vast room for legitimate disagreement about how these words should be interpreted. In effect, the courts become another forum for interested parties to clash over conflicting values and interests. Justice Rehnquist, for example, summarized the benzene controversy as follows: "I believe that this litigation presents the Court with what has to be one of the most difficult issues that could confront a decision maker: whether the statistical possibility of future deaths should ever be disregarded in light of the economic costs of preventing those deaths."[109]

In the case of "feasibility," the contending parties had no trouble finding their favored decision rule embodied in this word. To industrial interests, feasible meant capable of being done with costs reasonable in light of projected benefits. To Bingham and organized labor, feasible meant capable of being done without massive industrial disruption and loss of jobs. And to Justice Rehnquist the word was simply "a legislative mirage, appearing to some members [of Congress] but not to others, and assuming any form desired by the beholder." If the political complexion of the Court had been only slightly altered, an entirely different definition of feasibility might have emerged. Ambiguity about such a key phrase is perhaps an indication that any more precise legislative formulation of the limits of

OSHA's authority would have weakened or undermined the political consensus that created the agency in the first place.

The same point applies to the significant-risk doctrine, whose interpretation is likely to be a key issue in future regulatory controversies.[110] The fact that a significant risk is not self-defining means that the doctrine raises many more questions than it answers. "Significance" seems to imply that risk is a one-dimensional concept that can be subdivided into two categories—significant and insignificant. Our analyses of both formaldehyde and benzene suggest otherwise. Does significance refer to the severity of a suspected health effect (for example, leukemia versus reversible chromosome damage), or does it also account somehow for the number of persons exposed to the toxic substance? Is the potency of a carcinogen the dimension of concern, or does significance also account somehow for the quality of evidence (animal data versus human data, say) about carcinogenicity? Cancer risk is a multidimensional concept that is not comfortably or credibly collapsed into simple notions of significance.

Uncertainty about what Justice Stevens meant by significance can be seen as a strength of the Court's plurality opinion. Case law proceeds iteratively between enunciation of general doctrine and application to specific fact and policy situations. Over time, then, one can expect that federal agencies and reviewing courts will fashion a richer and more comprehensible doctrine of significant risk. That is arguably what has happened to the feasibility notion, where somewhat more specific ideas about what is technologically and economically feasible have emerged from litigation about prior OSHA standards.

Our view is that the Stevens opinion, even if saved by future evolution of the significant-risk doctrine, illustrates some dangers of judicial activism in this area. The ambiguity of "significant risk" in the plurality opinion may reflect the twin evils of ignorance and opportunism. It is quite possible (perhaps likely) that the justices and their law clerks did not comprehend the full scope of the problem they were addressing. Compounding this simplistic perception of the issues were the internal politics of the Court itself. Perhaps Stevens was guilty of what Rehnquist criticized Congress for doing with the word "feasible." By appealing to common-sense notions of "safe" and "significance," without offering precise formulations, Stevens attempted to marshal the votes of other justices on this highly controversial question. In cases where the plurality opinion does offer specific formulations, such as, the 1 in 1,000 guideline, the justices reveal their oversimplified view of the tasks of assessing and evaluating cancer risks.

Even if not inherently simplistic, "feasibility" and "significance" are both synthetic or integrative concepts. They presume some (usually unspecified) combination of factual, predictive, and evaluative contributions to decision making. This mixing of science, forecasting, and policy preference about standards is not very helpful in allocating accountable discretion among legislators, scientists, bureaucrats, and judges. A good solution to that problem requires, as we argue in Chapter 7, a more explicit decomposition of the regulator's decision problem.

The various decision rules, despite their apparent diversity, are actually quite limited and narrow in their approach to solving the problem. Only the significant-risk doctrine addresses priority setting and standard setting simultaneously, and it does so, as we have seen, in a highly elusive way. Moreover, all three doctrines approach standard setting by trying to answer the same simple question. How tightly should emissions or exposures to the suspected carcinogen be controlled by command-and-control regulation? A more comprehensive decision rule is needed for sound management of the entire problem of regulation.

5 · INTERPRETING THE SCIENTIFIC EVIDENCE ON BENZENE AND CANCER

BENZENE IS in many respects a classical chemical. It was discovered in 1825 by one of the era's preeminent chemists, Michael Faraday. Its chemical structure intrigued, evaded, and finally revealed itself to another prominent nineteenth-century chemist, Friedrich Kekule von Stradonitz in 1866. Benzene quickly found a place in many different industries as a versatile solvent, a fundamental unit in organic synthesis, and a component of fuels.

Benzene's volatility is the source of both its utility as a solvent and its hazardousness. As the liquid vaporizes, it migrates from the production process to the lungs of workers. By the late nineteenth century, it was clear that humans and animals exposed to benzene suffered damage to their bone marrow. Dose-dependent effects ranged in severity from a transient reduction in the number of blood cells produced by the bone marrow to a complete—and fatal—loss of viability of the marrow.[1]

Recognition of these effects, and the actions taken to mitigate them, followed a classic pattern. For the first few decades of the twentieth century, only a handful of physicians and industrial hygienists reported occasional fatalities caused by exposure to benzene in the workplace, and these exposures remained uncontrolled. Airborne concentrations of benzene in the workplace were rarely measured. What measurements there were revealed levels of from hundreds to thousands of ppm.

By the 1930s industrial hygienists generally had come to recognize that benzene was a hazard and began to set allowable upper limits for workers' exposure to benzene in air. The earliest limit, recommended in 1941, was 100 ppm. Over the decades the allowable upper limit was reduced to 50 ppm, then 35 ppm, then 25 ppm (see Table 5.1). As

This chapter was written with the assistance of Scott Wolff and Angela Boggs.

Table 5.1 Recommended limits for occupational exposure to benzene in air.

Year	Recommended standard
1941	100 ppm
1947	50 ppm 8-hour TWA
1948	35 ppm 8-hour TWA
1957	25 ppm 8-hour TWA
1963	25 ppm ceiling
1969	10 ppm 8-hour TWA
1971–present	10 ppm 8-hour TWA; 25 ppm acceptable ceiling; 50 ppm max. ceiling (10 min.)

Source: R. A. Rinsky, F. J. Young, and A. B. Smith, "Leukemia in Benzene Workers," *American Journal of Industrial Medicine,* 2 (1981): 217–245.

noted in Chapter 4, the current OSHA standard, adopted in 1971, is 10 ppm, on the basis of an eight-hour TWA; peak airborne levels of up to 25 ppm, and 50 ppm for 10 minutes, are also allowed.

The 1920s and 1930s saw the first reports of leukemia associated with exposure to benzene. A large number of clinical case reports and several epidemiological studies have followed. Although the information is not uniformly damning, there are so many positive human findings that the negative ones are unpersuasive. Benzene is considered one of the "known" human carcinogens, of which there are only about twenty.

Yet while its carcinogenicity has been well established, the biological mechanisms through which benzene causes leukemia remain largely undiscovered. There are estimates of how frequently the benzene-damaged bone marrow is transformed into a cancerous marrow, but there is no real understanding of why or how this transformation occurs, nor of how the process changes with changing levels of benzene exposure. The key problem is estimation of the risks associated with the relatively low levels of occupational exposure to benzene that currently prevail in the United States. Regulators need to know whether these levels present risks that should be reduced and controlled.

In this chapter we discuss both the clinical and case-report investigations that identified benzene as a human carcinogen and the epidemiological studies that have tried to quantify the risk. We then consider the evidence that benzene damages chromosomes, present the recent results of long-term bioassays of benzene in laboratory animals, and discuss alternative views of the mechanisms likely to play a role in the toxicity of benzene.

In all of this we see a rather unusual pattern of evidence: most of the data come directly from observations in humans. This is in sharp contrast to the cases of formaldehyde and many other chemicals, for which tests in laboratory animals have provided the sole or primary evidence of carcinogenicity. Yet while for the most part the problem of "mouse-to-man" extrapolation does not exist for benzene, there is still the problem of extrapolating from high doses of benzene—for which the strongest evidence for carcinogenicity obtains—to the lower doses workers encounter today. In both laboratory animal bioassays and epidemiologic investigations, it has been difficult to establish the effects of benzene at low doses. This limitation in the data has proven to be quite problematic for the standard-setting process.

In some cases the scientific community is polarized by deep underlying disagreements. Credible, indeed eminent, physicians and health scientists find themselves on opposite sides of important issues. For example, Donald Hunter—an eminent British physician, a student of benzene's toxicity since the late 1930s, and author of five editions of the classic text, *The Diseases of Occupations* (1955-1975)—writes, "The safe concentration of benzene vapor in a factory or workshop is ZERO parts per million" (emphasis in original).[1] On the other side, James Jandl, an eminent Harvard hematologist and acknowledged expert on bone marrow toxicity, believes there is a threshold for benzene-induced toxicity and leukemia, probably somewhat below 100 ppm, and certainly above 10 ppm.[2]

Those who argue that low exposure levels are safe note that benzene is different from most of the other human carcinogens, is not a mutagen, and has only very recently (and after much effort) been shown to be a carcinogen in laboratory animals. Benzene, they argue, is not a classical carcinogen, but rather is carcinogenic only through its effects as a bone marrow toxin. Because the toxic effects appear only after chronic exposure to high levels of benzene, benzene-induced leukemia is likely to be similarly dose dependent.

Further, it is argued, although benzene does appear to cause human leukemia, it does not appear to be a particularly *potent* leukemogen. This is a matter of some debate, of course, for the concept and definition of "potency" with respect to carcinogens are controversial. But both sides acknowledge that the fraction of a benzene-exposed population of workers that develops leukemia is very much smaller than the fraction of a population occupationally exposed to other known carcinogens—2-naphthylamine, for example—that develops cancer.

Those who argue that no level of benzene exposure is safe note that benzene has now been shown unequivocally to produce cancer in laboratory rats and mice at many different sites, including organs unrelated to the bone marrow or to leukemia. This, they argue, casts doubt on the notion that because there is a threshold for bone marrow toxicity there is also a threshold for benzene-induced cancer; the bone marrow may not be the only target organ in humans. Even if bone marrow is the only target, this camp claims that far too little is known about the genesis of leukemia—whether induced by benzene or by anything else—to be certain that a no-effects level exists.

To clarify the nature of this disagreement, it is necessary to take a careful look at the scientific evidence and how it has emerged.

▪ The Bone Marrow and Benzene

Terminology

Most of the elements of blood are formed in the bone marrow; the red blood cells (erythrocytes), the white blood cells (leukocytes), and the platelets (thrombocytes). There are several subclasses of leukocytes, the major ones being neutrophils and lymphocytes, both of which contribute to immune function.

Cytopenia ("penia" means "lack") refers to a diminution in the number of circulating blood cells in general; lymphocytopenia, thrombocytopenia, and so on refer to a lack of a specific type of cell. Anemia refers to a diminution in the number of red cells and/or in the amount of available hemoglobin. Cytopenias result from compromised function of the bone marrow, such as may result from exposure to myelotoxins ("myelo" refers to bone marrow) like benzene. Pancytopenia—the diminution of all types of blood cells—is thought to result from destruction of stem cells, which serve as a common progenitor of the different mature cell types. Severe toxicity to the marrow can result in aplastic anemia, a potentially fatal syndrome in which the cells of the marrow disappear, and blood cells are no longer formed at all. Leukemia, in contrast, is a cancer originating in the bone marrow, characterized by unchecked growth and proliferation of one or more types of transformed blood cells or their progenitors.

There are two major subtypes of leukemia: acute and chronic.

Acute leukemia involves an apparently uncontrolled proliferation of blast cells, which are immature, only partially differentiated blood cells. Acute myelogenous leukemia (AML) is both the most common type of leukemia in adults and the type most frequently associated with benzene. Myelogenous refers to blast cells in the myeloid cell line, which give rise to all of the blood cell types except lymphocytes. AML is therefore also referred to as acute nonlymphocytic leukemia, or ANLL. The long-term prognosis for patients with AML is currently extremely poor. Acute lymphocytic leukemia (ALL), in contrast, is predominantly a disease of children, although it may arise in individuals up to age forty. ALL in children, which is often quite responsive to chemotherapy, has not generally been associated with benzene.

Chronic myelogenous leukemia (CML) differs from AML in several aspects. Instead of uncontrolled predominance of a specific blast cell, CML is characterized by an increased number of myeloid cells at any stage of maturation. Chemotherapy can produce remissions of three or four years' duration, but CML then typically transforms itself into a syndrome very similar to, and as fatal as, AML. CML has occasionally been associated with exposures to benzene. Finally, chronic lymphocytic leukemia (CLL) is a slowly progressive, rarely fatal, disease of the elderly involving abnormal proliferation of lymphocytes. CLL has not generally been associated with benzene.

Clinical Studies

The first indications of morbidity and mortality associated with occupational exposures to benzene were reported in Sweden in 1897.[3] Nine young women employed in a tire factory using benzene-based rubber cement hemorrhaged from various sites; four of them died. All of the women were found to be anemic; their blood was lacking in platelets (thrombocytopenic) and almost totally lacking in white cells (leucopenic). Similar cases were reported in the United States in the first two decades of this century.[4] Two fatalities caused by hemorrhaging were reported among men who operated a fabric-coating machine. According to the case report, "The company had made tests of the air around the coating machines, for it was anxious to prevent the escape of the solvent, which it was trying to recover and use again. Something less than 5 per cent (50,000 ppm) was reported to be the highest concentration of benzene found in the air, and it is evident that the officials considered this amount too little to cause any anxiety."[5] The report mentions that airborne levels on the order of 100 ppm were considered at the time to be quite small, although this investigator and some others felt that the "marked susceptibility of certain individuals" might put some at risk of injury even at these levels.

Soon thereafter the first reports appeared linking leukemia to benzene exposure. In 1928 acute lymphoblastic leukemia was reported in a French worker who had been exposed for about five years.[6] By 1938 some ten cases of leukemia related to benzene exposure had been reported world-wide.[7] Two more cases apparently resulted from chronic benzene exposure in factories near Boston.[8]

Enrico Vigliani and his coworkers, clinical hematologists in Milan, spent the next several decades treating and studying workers with hematologic disease and histories of exposure to benzene. They reported on 83 cases of benzene-related blood diseases among workers who had sought and received compensation in Milan and Pavia in the 1960s. Of the 83 workers, 50 were still alive and anemic by the mid-1970s, 14 had died of aplastic anemia, and 19 had died of leukemia.[9]

Vigliani's work led to the banning of benzene as a solvent for glues and inks in Italy in the mid-1960s, as well as to the replacement of benzene with toluene as a solvent in the Italian rotogravure industry. Ten years later Vigliani and Forni reported that they had seen "no new cases of aplastic anemia, nor of leukemia." They also noted that "toluene-exposed workers do not show the chromosome aberrations frequently seen in workers exposed to benzene."[10]

The Italian work was paralleled in Turkey by Muzaffer Aksoy, a clinical hematologist who studied benzene-induced diseases among shoe workers, of whom there are reportedly some 30,000 in Istanbul. Prior to 1955 or so, Turkish shoemakers apparently mixed their own glues by working together rubber and gasoline. By about 1960, however, commercially prepared, benzene-based adhesives became available and were widely used. Aksoy reported the consequences:

Thereafter, since 1961, cases of aplastic anemia started to occur gradually. Until 1972 we collected 34 cases of aplastic anemia with long-term exposure to benzene. Furthermore, an investigation was carried out in Istanbul on 217 normal appearing workers manufacturing shoes with solvents containing benzene under unhygienic conditions. In 51 of them (23.5%) hematological abnormalities consisting of leucopenia, thrombocytopenia, pancytopenia, pseudo-Pelger anomaly, etc. attributed to benzene exposure, were detected. Since 1967, numerous cases of leukemia were found in the same work places where outbreaks of the benzene poisoning or hematological abnormalities have been observed.[11]

The use of benzene-based glues was banned in Turkey in the late 1960s. By the mid-1970s Aksoy reported that the incidence of leukemia among shoe workers had declined markedly.[12]

There is widespread agreement that these clinical case reports and later epidemiologic studies are sufficient to put benzene on the list of known human carcinogens.[13] But there are marked disagreements over the quantitative questions.[14] Is a worker exposed to benzene twice as likely as a nonexposed worker to die of leukemia? Twenty times as likely? What levels and durations of exposure to benzene result in what levels of risk?

On the methodological level there is debate about what kinds of human studies can best provide the basis for such estimates. Aksoy and Vigliani provided a series of clinical case reports, not carefully designed epidemiological investigations of an entire cohort of benzene-exposed workers or case-control studies. Typically the clinical case reporters and the analytical epidemiologists disagree about the utility of information generated by each other's approach. These disagreements are especially relevant here, because the two groups tend to draw very different conclusions about benzene.

The clinical case reporters contend that their observational studies have one unarguable advantage over large epidemiological studies of mortality: they study live patients, not death certificates. Clinicians can study each case in depth, take detailed and repeated histories of each patient, and watch the progression or regression of disease. They can thus estimate the consequences of specific exposures in ways that an investigator tallying diagnoses from a large number of death certificates is unable to do. Among other things, clinical case reporters are able to make reasonably reliable estimates of latency periods. (Vigliani identified latency periods ranging from one to forty years between onset of benzene exposure and onset of leukemia. Aksoy estimated latencies to be from one to fifteen years.) Case reporters also believe that a hematologist who sees twenty cases of leukemia in a single decade among benzene-exposed workers and sees no cases or only one or two in the next decade among toluene-exposed workers has strong evidence that benzene causes leukemia and that toluene does not. Assuming that the sets of workers are of roughly comparable size, some clinicians are even willing to use such evidence to argue that previous occupational exposures to benzene caused a ten- to twentyfold increase in risk of leukemia.

On the other hand, epidemiologists note that clinical studies often do not last long enough or encompass large enough changes in exposure to allow for such comparisons. And they argue that the clinicians have no way of determining what would have happened to those workers in the absence of exposures to benzene, because case reports do not include concurrent examination of large numbers of unexposed controls. The case reporters can count the number of published cases of benzene-induced leukemias—150 according to one estimate,[15] 250 according to another.[16] But they cannot calculate rates or relative risks because they do not know how many workers have been exposed, whether they have an accurate count of all the relevant cases, or how many leukemias would have been expected among those cohorts had they not been exposed to benzene.

All calculations of relative risk are somewhat disputable, since they assume that carcinogenic risks operate multiplicatively not additively, as we discuss in Chapter 6. Determining relative risk according to conventional methods requires two incidence rates, one on the exposed group and another in some control population. The former divided by the latter equals the relative risk.

Case reporters have made some relative risk calculations. They obtain the numerator by dividing the observed number of cases by some estimate of the exposed population, and the denominator from the local or national rates recorded in cancer registries. Vigliani and Saita, for example, used an estimate of the annual incidence of acute leukemia in the general population of Milan (1 per 20,000) as a denominator.[17] From this and their case reports they calculated that benzene-exposed workers were at a relative risk of 20 for developing acute leukemia. Aksoy allowed readers to construct their own ratios. He calculated that the annual incidence of leukemia among Turkish shoe workers was 13 per 100,000 and stated that the annual incidence in the general population was 6 per 100,000.[18] In his 1977 risk assessment, Richard Wilson, a risk assessor and professor of physics at Harvard, used these numbers and calculated a relative risk of 2.[19]

The question of what rate to use is a tricky one in the absence of good data. As we discuss in Chapter 6, by using different data and assumptions, one can reach very different results. For example, the total leukemia rate can be adjusted by omitting the lymphoid leukemias (on the presumption that benzene produces only myelogenous leukemias) and by adjusting for age. In this way, a rate for myelogenous leukemia in Turkey of only 0.66 per 100,000 was calculated for use in one EPA risk assessment.[20] If one uses Aksoy's figures for the numerator and EPA's for the denominator, the relative risk becomes 20—ten times Wilson's original estimate.

Many epidemiologists maintain that the denominator cannot be assumed or derived informally from some national or even regional statistic, but must be observed in concurrently studied, nonexposed controls. There is no guarantee, they argue, that the experiences of nonexposed workers will follow some average population rate, as Otto Wong discovered in a recently completed epidemiological investigation of benzene-exposed workers. That retrospective cohort study found 7 leukemias among some 4,600 benzene-exposed chemical workers, while 6.0 cases would have been expected based upon incidence rates for the general U.S. population. Concurrently, some 3,000 chemical workers who were not exposed to benzene were studied as controls. In the latter group 3.4 cases would have been expected but no cases were observed![21] Neither Wong nor his invited reviewers could account for this discrepancy.[22] Does it mean that chemical workers for some reason have lower than normal leukemia rates, or is this unlikely outcome simply the result of chance? While some analysts offered calculations (with various assumptions) of relative risks based on this data, others were more impressed both by the shakiness of such calculations in this case and by the more general problem it highlights of selecting an appropriate reference rate.

Finally, some analysts are critical of both clinical and epidemiological studies because of the lack of knowledge of workers' real exposure. These critics note that information about the levels and patterns of benzene exposure experienced by any of the subjects studied has ranged from nonexistent to sketchy and conjectural. In fact, obtaining such information would require making analytical chemical measurements and assumptions about exposure-dose relationships, both of which physicians typically are neither equipped to make nor particularly interested in.

• Epidemiological Studies

There is agreement that both epidemiological studies and case reports have shown that in the past, relatively high exposures to benzene in the workplace caused deaths from aplastic anemia and leukemia. There is disagreement over whether current, relatively low, exposures in American workplaces continue to cause workers' deaths. The disagreement arises in part because of the relative infrequency of the diseases and the often long latency period between exposure to the chemical and clinical signs of leukemia. Thus one cannot determine whether a case of leukemia found, for example, in a sixty-year-old rubber worker during 1982 was caused by exposure to benzene in 1980 or in 1960 (or perhaps, though less likely, not by benzene by all). This conundrum has important implications for policymaking. The recommended limits of exposure to benzene were halved around 1970, and many maintain that it may be too early to tell what difference this has made.

This is in striking contrast to the situations studied by Vigliani in Italy and Aksoy in Turkey. Workers in those countries had been exposed apparently to hundreds of ppm of benzene and many cases of leukemia were noted. After benzene was banned for most uses, within a decade the incidence of leukemia among groups of workers exposed to toluene and other substitutes for benzene diminished dramatically. In contrast, the benzene-exposed American workers were refiners and rubber workers, not shoemakers; they were exposed over the last several decades to tens, not hundreds, of ppm of benzene; and they are now exposed to less benzene, but not to none.

Another interpretive problem is that leukemia is a relatively low-frequency event, so that minor fluctuations or trends in the leukemia rate over time are not detectable. Indeed the age-adjusted death rate for leukemia in the U.S. population appears not to have changed between 1950 and 1980. There are, furthermore, at least two opposing temporal trends in benzene exposure: occupational standards have been steadily declining over the century (and with them, presumably, individual occupational exposures), but production of benzene in the United States has increased substantially, especially since World War II, which presumably means that *environmental* exposures to benzene have risen.

Regardless of the extent to which benzene is an underlying cause of leukemia in the U.S. population, then, it is not clear what we can learn from temporal trends in leukemia death rates, or even leukemia incidence rates.

The Study by Infante and Coworkers

The first—and still most controversial—retrospective mortality study of benzene-exposed workers in the U.S. was performed by Peter Infante and others at NIOSH.[23] As was explained in Chapter 4 this study was prominent in the 1977 attempt by OSHA to lower the occupational benzene standard. It remains important because one of the original researchers has published a reconstruction of benzene exposure levels in the two factories studied and then used these estimates as a basis for a quantitative risk assessment.[24]

Infante and coworkers studied workers who had been occupationally exposed to benzene in the manufacture of a rubber product called Pliofilm. The study cohort included all white males who had been employed in the production of Pliofilm at either of two factories in Ohio any time during the decade of the 1940s and who were still alive at the end of that decade. At the time of the first report in 1977, the mortality status of only 75 percent of the cohort had been determined. Of the 140 deaths, 7 were caused by leukemia, compared to the 1.4 or 1.5 that would have been expected.[25] Many epidemiologists were critical of the researchers for publishing the report before at least 90 percent of the cohort had been accounted for, which is the more usual practice. (As it happened, a second report, with more than 90 percent of the cohort accounted for, found essentially the same ratio of observed to expected leukemia deaths. And a third report found the same results with 98 percent follow-up.)[26]

Infante and coworkers were quite clear about their own policy position on benzene. In introducing the study, they wrote: "In the 50 years since the first reported case of benzene-associated leukemia, benzene has been neither widely acknowledged nor uniformly controlled as a carcinogen in the U.S. The failure to control benzene as a carcinogen has resulted primarily from the reluctance of industry and Government to accept the accumulated case-reports and epidemiological observations as scientific evidence of the leukaemogenic properties of benzene."[27] In discussing the study's conclusions, they stated: "We hope that our findings, which demonstrate overwhelmingly an increased risk of leukemia in workers exposed to benzene, will stimulate efforts to control occupational and consumer exposure to benzene, an agent known for almost a century to be a powerful bone-marrow poison."[28]

Private consultants Tabershaw and Lamm criticized the design, reporting, and conclusions of the Infante group's study. In particular they claimed that the researchers knew that a leukemia cluster existed before the study began: "A local newspaper had investigated the cluster of leukemia cases in pliofilm manufacturing and reported the findings in detail in April and May, 1976, while Infante et al. were collecting their cohort. All leukemia cases in cohort A (the only one with cases of acute myelogenous leukemia) had been seen by the chief hematologist at the local hospital who had been professionally and legally concerned about this cluster for more than 10 years."[29] Infante's group countered: "The study cohort was selected before we knew of any case of leukemia among pliofilm production workers at either locality. Subsequently, a newspaper in locality A became aware of our study and started an investigation of its own resulting in its identification of leukemia among benzene-exposed workers, some of whom were former pliofilm production workers. In June, 1977, during routine ascertainment of pathology reports for the leukemia cases, a hematologist in locality A informed us of several previously identified cases of leukemia among workers at that location."[30]

Six years later, Lamm and Wilson appeared to be unconvinced by the results of Infante's work. They were also forthright about their opinions regarding the regulation of benzene: "The authors became interested in the problems of benzene exposure when . . . OSHA . . . proposed in 1977 to change the occupational standard for benzene exposure to 1 ppm from 10 ppm. It seemed to the authors that OSHA had presented no good reason for the proposed new level."[31] In apparent reference to Infante and coworkers' study, Lamm and Wilson suggested: "If we see a large apparent effect of the type we are looking for in one particular plant and then decide to make a study, examining that plant, the resultant epidemiological study would find a spuriously high effect. The best procedure in such circumstances is to study . . . other . . . factories."[32] In other words, they argue, if an investigator sets out to study a previously identified cancer cluster—that is, a number of cancer cases that appear to be unusually grouped, either spatially or temporally— then he will by definition find an unusually high frequency of cancers.

From a policy perspective the critical issue is whether the cluster of cancers was actually *caused* by the occupational benzene exposures. If it was, one could generalize the results of this study to all workers similarly exposed to benzene. Alternatively, the cluster could be the result of some other aspect of the factory and its workers, including random variation—in which case one could not so generalize. If there are enough cases and enough exposure data to establish a dose-response relationship *within* the cluster, then one can be more confident that the association is not spurious. Otherwise, one has to look to studies of other workers exposed to benzene for confirmation of the association.

The Other Studies

About ten other groups of epidemiologists have studied benzene-exposed workers. The studies have all been plagued, to a greater or lesser degree, with similar problems: low incidences of leukemia among both controls and study populations; unknown or incomplete work histories of subjects and controls; poorly characterized, often mixed, exposures to benzene and other chemicals; and uncertain validity of the diagnoses of leukemia subtypes. Interpretations of the studies, therefore, are beset by caveats and various disagreements.

At issue is the shape of the dose-response curve, especially at relatively low doses. The controversy persists in part because the studies have not reached the same conclusions. The smaller studies tend to be positive (with relative risks roughly comparable to those reported by Infante and coworkers), but the larger ones tend to be negative. And this technical ambiguity does not occur in a vacuum. Investigators, critics, and policy makers are all aware of the scientific history and the policy context. An epidemiologist setting out to study "the benzene problem" is cognizant both of the fifty-year history of case reports and of the current disagreements. That is what makes the problem interesting. He or she inevitably holds some prior beliefs as to benzene's leukemogenicity. This is not to say that the new studies are necessarily biased by the old, only that this is not virgin territory.

Furthermore, differences among study results tend to be magnified and exaggerated, and their proponents and critics are polarized by attempts to use the studies to support various positions concerning the assessment of safe levels and the setting of appropriate standards. In the absence of regulatory imperatives, most clinicians and epidemiologists, who are generally too self-conscious about the limitations of their studies, would be uncomfortable with the use of their data in quantitative risk assessments. But given the pressure placed on scientists by the regulatory process, an agnostic or cautious stance is often difficult to maintain.

The associate medical director of Exxon, J. J. Thorpe, was the first to undertake a large-scale investigation of workers who might have been exposed to benzene. He is as forthright as Infante and coworkers about his interest: "The comments by an official of a European government agency that data from medical records of a company such as Exxon might influence their action in recommending a ceiling limit on benzene provided the incentive for undertaking this study."[33]

Thorpe observed 18 leukemia deaths among his study group. By his calculations, 23 would have been expected. He also estimated a semiquantitative index of subjects' exposure to benzene, which did not correlate with the incidence of leukemia. He concluded "that low levels of potential benzene exposure are unrelated to leukemia mortality." He did allow that there was a slight preponderance of "observed" over "expected" deaths in the subgroup of workers classified (by their job descriptions) as being potentially exposed to liquids containing 1 percent or more of benzene, but this did not enter into his conclusions.

Steven Brown, at Berkeley, was critical of Thorpe's report, questioning both its origins and its conclusions: "Without hoping to be able to comment objectively upon the possible bias or motivation of an associate director of one of the world's largest petroleum companies . . . I should like to . . . question . . . the reliability of the number of 'observed' or reported cases of leukemia among Exxon workers."[34] Brown suggested that this number might well be an underestimate if workers left the company before being diagnosed. Thorpe countered that the Exxon work force was very stable and that leukemia cases among nonemployed controls might have been *underreported*.[35] These are exactly the kinds of judgmental issues that are difficult to resolve on purely scientific grounds.

There are also disagreements about how the data are to be analyzed and interpreted. Another epidemiologist, Otto Wong, who has performed a large study of benzene-exposed workers, commented that Thorpe's "benzene-exposed employees experienced a two-fold risk of leukemia when compared to non-exposed employees."[36] This comparison makes the study appear to be more positive than Thorpe's interpretations indicated, but Wong did not say clearly whether he believed that the comparison he mentioned is valid. He noted that it would be inappropriate to compare the two standardized mortality ratios if they derived from populations with different age distributions. He noted also that Thorpe's data do not allow one to compute those age distributions directly. The average ages of death of leukemia cases in both populations were essentially the same, however, which suggests similar age distributions. Again, which methods for summarizing the data are appropriate and how should one interpret such results?

Rushton and Alderson of the Institute of Cancer Research in Great Britain also conducted a major study, investigating mortality patterns among workers in eight oil refineries. No overall excess of leukemia deaths appeared; 30 cases were observed when 32 were expected. When the cases were stratified according to whether the individuals had sustained "low," "medium," or "high" exposures to benzene, there did appear to be "an increase in the risk of leukemia in the groups whose exposure to benzene was assessed as medium or high." The authors are not particularly alarmed by this: "If there were an increased risk of leukemia due to benzene exposure, it could have only been one that affected a very small proportion of men within the refinery workforce."[37]

Wong's study of more than 7,500 chemical workers (4,600 of whom were exposed to benzene) is among the studies most subject to divergent interpretation. As mentioned previously, the most outstanding result was not the number of leukemia deaths among those exposed (7 cases were observed while 6 were expected), but the complete absence of leukemia deaths among the unexposed workers (when 3.4 cases were expected). Wong apparently regards the results of his study as somewhat equivocal, but on balance positive. He concluded:

In spite of limitations, this study has demonstrated that chemical workers occupationally exposed to benzene experienced significant mortality excess from leukemia, as well as the broader category of all lymphatic and hematopoietic cancer, when compared to chemical workers who were not occupationally exposed to benzene . . . The data further show significant dose-response relationships between cumulative benzene exposure and excess mortality from leukemia . . . The shape of the dose-response curve was less definite, due to the variability of the available data."[38]

Some of Wong's critics are hesitant to draw conclusions from the study, even though they are impressed by the quantity and quality of his work. Brian MacMahon, professor of epidemiology at Harvard, for example, wrote that Wong "has done an excellent job of analysis and reporting of what is essentially a weak data base . . . It seems doubtful to me that this cohort will ever add anything to existing knowledge that will be biologically meaningful or that will influence the regulatory process. The numbers are too small and the non-exposed group too unusual—for reasons that I do not understand."[39]

Similar disagreements surround the much smaller study by Ott and coworkers of workers at the Dow Chemical Corporation. But in this case it is the authors who have been reluctant to draw conclusions from their data, while their critics have argued that the results implicate low-level exposure to benzene as leukemogenic. The epidemiologists found 71 deaths among a cohort of 594 workers exposed to benzene in a Dow plant. Of these deaths 5 "were judged to be of clinical interest with regard to benzene toxicity." One death was caused by pernicious anemia, one by aplastic anemia, and 3 by leukemia. The authors calculated that only 0.8 leukemia deaths were to be expected. They noted that this excess is statistically significant ($p <$ .047), but they shied away from implicating benzene as a cause of the excess, stating: "In these cases, varied work histories and the lack of medical history made a retrospective assessment of the possible relationship to benzene exposure very judgmental."[40] The authors estimated cumulative benzene exposures for each worker and found no correlation between these estimated exposures and the observed leukemia cases. Given the small number of cases, however, they and others agree that it would be difficult to detect any such correlation.

Other analysts have been impressed by exactly what the investigators were unimpressed by. The three individuals who died of leukemia were apparently exposed to low (2–9 ppm TWA) or very low (less than 2 ppm TWA) exposures to benzene. Ott's group took this to mean that benzene was not likely to have been the leukemogen in these cases. Infante and White, however, interpreted it to mean that even low levels of benzene were apparently leukemogenic.[41]

There is also disagreement over whether three was in fact the "correct" number of leukemia deaths in the cohort. Some argued that it ought to be two, since the death certificates for the third case listed pneumonia as the primary cause of death, with myeloblastic leukemia noted as another "significant condition."[42] Regardless of which number is correct, it is still very small. Some epidemiologists do not even calculate risk ratios for fewer than five cases, as a matter of general interpretive caution. And for this particular study, many have contended that quantitative interpretation is unwarranted.[43]

The question remains why different investigators choose to present their results as they do. Ott and coworkers summarized their findings in part, "No mortalities directly attributable to benzene exposure were observed."[44] The statement is strictly speaking, true, but what findings would justify direct attribution? After all, no epidemiological study can provide such "direct attribution"—as the tobacco industry is fond of pointing out.

The role of an investigator's judgment in characterizing such results is clearly illustrated by contrasting the conclusion of Ott's study with that presented in another mortality study of benzene-exposed workers in which similar numbers of leukemia deaths were observed. In the latter study, researchers from the University of Arizona and the National Cancer Institute observed 3 deaths from leukemia where they expected 0.44. The investigators summarized their results as follows: "The findings are consistent with previous reports of leukemia following occupational exposure to benzene."[45]

One of the largest epidemiological studies, recently completed, illustrates the same point. Workers at two Shell Oil Company plants (Wood River and Deer Park) were found to have an excess number of deaths from AML. Philip Cole, an eminent cancer epidemiologist at the University of Alabama, was hired by Shell to review and evaluate the study. He concluded:

From the years 1973 through 1982 there was an approximately four-fold increased risk of death due to AML among men employed at Wood River in comparison to men in the United States general population . . . *As to 1983 and later, there is some reason to believe that the problem will continue* [emphasis added]. There is no reasonable possibility that the data are the result of any error or errors or random variations of consequence; nor is it likely that these findings can be attributed to confounding by a non-occupational cause of AML.

The specific cause of the excess of AML at Wood River is unknown. However, benzene is an established cause of AML, and there is anecdotal evidence that in years past benzene was present in the ambient air at Wood River at levels that exceed the current standard. Thus, benzene is the most likely cause of the excesses seen. Nonetheless, the possibility remains that some other occupational exposure or exposures, alone or in combination, are culpable.[46]

In contrast, R. E. Joyner, corporate medical director at Shell, phrased the conclusions of the same study somewhat differently:

The initial review of the data has not identified areas of concern with respect to current health risks. Data on leukemia at two of the five locations did warrant further study. The results of more detailed studies indicate that at one of the five refineries, Wood River, Illinois, mortality rates for one form of leukemia, acute myeloid, was higher than normal. Also an excess of acute myeloid leukemia observed at Deer Park, Texas Refinery, while not statistically significant, raises questions which require additional studies. However, at both of these locations, total cancer-related deaths were normal and *we have no reason to conclude that a leukemia risk currently exists at any of our refinery locations."* (emphasis added).[47]

Interpreted in certain ways, these statements are not necessarily contradictory. Joyner did not rule out the possibility, for example, that benzene could have increased AML rates in the past. But the two statements clearly differ in their emphases and in their summaries of the evidence.

At Wood River, 14 leukemia deaths were observed; 6.6 were expected. Deer Park had 6 leukemia deaths; 2.6 were expected. In particular, 8 AML deaths occurred among workers at Wood River, while 2 were expected. Cole characterized these increases as "highly statistically significant" and commented: "At present, I remain of the persuasion that the most likely cause of the leukemias is benzene . . . Common sense tells me it's benzene, but you can't establish scientific fact on that."[48] Furthermore, Cole felt that the available data suggested that workers with leukemia were "more heavily exposed" to benzene than nonafflicted coworkers.

Perhaps not surprisingly, the Shell executive's interpretation differs.[49] Joyner stated that "there was no apparent difference in [workplace] benzene exposure levels between those who died of leukemia and those who didn't." He concluded that the study "produced no distinctly positive result, not even for benzene." Again, it is the fundamental, irreducible ambiguity of almost all epidemiological results, and the unavoidable role of judgment in interpreting them, that results in such divergent accounts of the same data.

Estimating Dose-Response Relationships

As noted above, a number of investigators have attempted to determine whether, within a given benzene-exposed cohort, those who developed leukemia were exposed to relatively higher levels of benzene than those who did not develop the disease. Strong evidence of such an association has not emerged, and this makes it worth asking about the sensitivity of such analyses.

The fact is that only a small fraction of those exposed to benzene at present levels develop leukemia. This leaves great room for a wide variety of genetic and environmental factors—essentially all unknown—to influence whether they develop the disease. More important, since there are always relatively few cases of this rare disease even in the largest studies, it is unlikely that stratification according to estimated levels of past exposure will reveal a dose-response relationship. The possibility of error, or "noise," in the relationship because of random variation is too great. In addition, assessments of past exposure are at best rough estimates, uninformed either by much actual data or by knowledge of underlying mechanisms of leukemia causation. Thus any stratification is likely to have mistakes that will obscure the actual relationship.

Further, it is not at all clear how to quantify exposures in order to best estimate the toxicologically significant doses. Data on workplace exposures are most often reported as eight-hour TWAs. Implicit in this expression is the assumption that the average level is the most appropriate measure of dose and, therefore, of toxicological response. It assumes that three workers all exposed to 1 ppm of benzene on a TWA basis are at equal risk, even though the first may be exposed to 1 ppm throughout the working day, the second exposed to 8 ppm for one hour and an undetectably low level for the other seven hours, and the third exposed to 48 ppm for ten minutes and essentially none for the rest of the day. But there is considerable debate about whether the average exposure level is the best measure of dose, or whether higher or "peak" exposures, even for correspondingly shorter durations, are more important because they are more likely to result in adverse health consequences. If peak exposure is the best measure, then data on how many workers are exposed to a given TWA level are unlikely to be completely informative.

Richard Irons of CIIT has generated some evidence to suggest that intermittent exposures are far more toxic.[50] He found that one particular benzene metabolite, hydroquinone, can induce what appears to be aplastic anemia in experimentally exposed mice. Continuous exposure, however, was not particularly effective. Producing aplastic anemia required intermittent exposures, even to considerably smaller total amounts. Drawing an analogy between the metabolite and some cancer chemotherapeutic agents, Irons hypothesized that hydroquinone attacks cells only in the midst of cell division, while resting stem cells are immune. His suggestion is that cells which remain dormant and therefore resistant in the presence of hydroquinone become active in its absence and so become vulnerable to its reintroduction.

This possibility is obviously very important for regulatory policy. It suggests that the low and relatively constant environmental exposures with which EPA is concerned may be of very limited consequence. In contrast, occupational exposure standards that significantly reduce allowable peak exposures might be more productive than those that strive merely to lower the TWA. Yet as the previous chapter described, the last eight years of effort to change the benzene standard have focused almost entirely on changing the TWA from 10 ppm to 1 ppm. This effort may well be beside the point if Irons's views of mechanism prove to be correct. In fact, OSHA's 1985 proposal to lower the TWA but remove all limits on short-term exposure could prove to be exactly the wrong approach!

Benzene producers themselves have noted the toxicological importance of transient high exposures to benzene. An Exxon report stated that although the current OSHA ceiling is 25 ppm, "individual companies . . . have adopted a 10 ppm ceiling (15 minute) limit to reduce excursions."[51] (They explain that the lower ceiling is based in part upon the "uncertainty regarding potential reproductive effects," which is odd, because nothing in the literature suggests that workplace exposures to benzene might be harmful to reproduction). And a report by Shell and British Petroleum speculates that "exposure to high concentrations is crucial in determining the onset of leukemia," although no supporting references are provided.[52]

Given the difficulties surrounding attempts to assess current exposures, it is no surprise that retrospective reconstruction of benzene exposures is problematic and controversial. Not only does no one know what the numbers mean, no one knows for the most part what the numbers were! Everyone agrees that in the past exposures were "high." Certainly benzene is a highly volatile compound, and the unguarded use of it in poorly ventilated work spaces—presumably the norm several decades ago—could easily have resulted in airborne levels in the range of several hundreds to a thousand or more ppm. The occasional measurements made decades ago seem to support this general supposition. But once analysts attempt to pick the most probable exposure levels associated with increased incidence of leukemia, the disagreements begin.

At issue is the potency of benzene as a leukemogen. Suppose one analyst speculates that historical workplace exposures averaging, say, 100 ppm were responsible for a given number of leukemia cases, while another analyst supposes that exposures averaging 400 ppm generated that number of leukemias. The first analyst would in effect be considering benzene four times more potent than the second analyst claims. Claims and counterclaims abound on this point: one group is charged with deflating the historical exposures, and hence inflating the attendant risks, while a second group is suspected by the first of inflating those exposures in order to deflate the risks.[53]

Epidemiology According to Types of Exposure

Some evidence of dose-response relationships does emerge when the various conflicting epidemiological studies on benzene are analyzed together. As we have seen, some studies of benzene-exposed workers have been positive and some have been negative. As a general matter, this is not particularly surprising: different studies of apparently similar populations often have opposite outcomes, most often because the sizes of the study populations differ substantially, and thus the investigations have differing powers.

In the case of benzene, however, the situation is not what might have been expected. Here the small studies have generally been positive and the large ones negative. Such a pattern of results might mean that benzene has not in fact been demonstrated to be a human leukemogen. Alternatively, it might mean that the various study populations are qualitatively and quantitatively different. It might be, for example, that the manner and extent to which different populations of benzene-exposed workers are exposed is crucial.

In the early positive case reports, all of the subjects were exposed to benzene in open workplace settings: making tires with benzene-based cements, working with open fabric-coating machines, using benzene-based inks and glues, or otherwise in intimate contact with benzene-based glues and vapors.

The positive epidemiologic studies appear to involve somewhat similar situations. The Pliofilm workers studied by Infante and co-workers operated a complex manufacturing process that required large quantities of pure benzene. The process was apparently very open until about 1946 and essentially closed thereafter. The excess leukemia deaths were observed among those who had made Pliofilm in the years between 1940 and 1950.

Consider too the benzene exposures at the small plant studied by Decoufle and coworkers, where workers manufactured chemical derivatives of benzene between 1947 and 1960. The plant processed some six million gallons of benzene annually. The processes were continuous—which is to say essentially closed—but the authors of the study noted that there were "multiple fugitive emissions peculiar to past process technology." They added:

In addition to exposures that resulted from day-to-day contact with the process itself, another source of benzene exposure originated from habits developed by individual workers. For example, according to union officials, it had been common practice for some workers to clean their hands, clothing, and tools with benzene. Furthermore, it was mentioned that some workers would siphon off benzene for home use. Although we recognize that these reports are anecdotal in nature, they do suggest that at least some workers received benzene exposures that were in excess of levels given off by the "ordinary run" of the manufacturing processes.[54]

The results of this study were also positive, although less strikingly so than those of Infante and coworkers. Their results were very similar to those of Ott's study of Dow Chemical workers, and the occupational settings were also very similar.

Contrast this with the processes studied and the results obtained by Thorpe at Exxon and by Rushton and Alderson. These groups studied petroleum refiners, whose exposures to benzene are qualitatively and quantitatively different from those of the above-mentioned groups. For one thing, petroleum contains only a low percentage of benzene. For another, the processes are not only continuous and closed, but also take place largely out-of-doors. And there are few, if any, opportunities for the "benzene abuse" described in the chemical manufacturing study above. These studies covered many more workers—thousands, instead of the hundreds studied by Infante, Decoufle, or Ott—but they simply were not exposed to much benzene, either in the distant or the more recent past. The negative results of Thorpe and of Rushton and Alderson say a lot about the relative safety of petroleum refining, but considerably less about safety or hazards of occupational benzene exposures.

Two studies are not consistent with the synthesis just offered, and both are difficult to interpret. The first is the positive study of Shell oil refinery workers. The results of the company's extensive, reconstructive exposure assessment for the two plants at which excess leukemia cases deaths occurred are inconclusive. A number of operations appeared to involve larger exposures to benzene than expected, but in general these were *not* the operations in which leukemia cases were found.

The second exception is Wong's large study of chemical workers, which, as noted above, had even more enigmatic results. Benzene-exposed workers died of leukemia at about the same rate as the general population. There were, however, considerably more leukemia deaths among the exposed workers than among the nonexposed worker controls, but this relative excess was due to an inexplicable deficit in leukemia deaths among the controls. Only with considerable subjective judgment can any conclusions concerning benzene exposures and leukemia be drawn from such results.

Unfortunately, judgmental reconciliations of apparently conflicting results tell us very little about the central policy issue: namely, the dose-response relationship at lower exposure levels. The available result, which is that "more seems worse," cannot credibly be stretched to provide the more precise estimates that some regulatory agencies are demanding.

▪ Chromosomal Damage and Mutations

Leukemia and anemias are not the only adverse health effects ascribable to benzene. Several studies have suggested that benzene has caused chromosomal damage in exposed workers. This is a very contentious issue, with both the measure of such effects and their significance much in dispute. Many different kinds of chromosomal changes—breaks in the chromosomes, chromosome rearrangements, exchanges between "sister" chromatids, and others—fall under the rubric of "chromosome damage." Further, different investigators have different methods for identifying and enumerating these aberrations. And almost nothing is known about the mechanisms of these alterations or their toxicological significance. The question is what functional consequences correspond to the various kinds of damage. Health effects could range from none through birth defects and cancer.

There is currently no evidence that the chromosomal damage induced by benzene produces adverse functional changes. But such evidence would be very difficult to obtain. Therefore the seriousness ascribed by investigators to chromosomal damage tends to depend in part upon their views about possible—as opposed to demonstrable—risks.

In 1978 OSHA regarded the chromosome-damaging ability of benzene to be of less concern than its leukemogenicity, but still serious.

While the record clearly demonstrated that benzene causes chromosomal aberrations, it is equally clear that there is no unanimity of opinion as to what the benzene-induced chromosome aberrations mean in terms of demonstrable health effects . . . It is also clear that for man, no quantitative dose-response relationship has been established for these effects. It is OSHA's interpretation of these findings that chromosomal damage represents an adverse biological event of serious concern which may pose or reflect a potential health risk and as such, must be considered in the larger purview of adverse health effects associated with benzene.[55]

Some arguments presented to OSHA stressed the potential seriousness of benzene-induced chromosomal changes, and another argument minimized it. The arguments of the first sort were that "while breaks may be repaired and are not necessarily mutational events (in the sense of being inherited), each occurrence increases the probability of a structural aberration, and therefore of a mutation"; and "because changes in the genes and chromosomes do not usually produce an immediate health hazard, they may go undetected for a lifetime or even for several generations. Yet, the human gene pool can become insidiously polluted."[56] On the other side, some analysts argued that benzene-induced chromosomal damage is unrelated to leukemia. OSHA accepted this but held that chromosomal damage might be either harmful per se or harmful through mechanisms unrelated to leukemogenesis.

The tentative nature of this scientific discussion might have kept it out of the regulatory process entirely, except for one salient feature: chromosomal damage occurs at very low levels of benzene exposure. And the question of whether "health effects" occur at such low levels is, as we have seen, at the center of the standard-setting debate.

At the time of OSHA's 1978 rulemaking on benzene, chromosomal damage in blood cells of workers exposed to high levels of benzene had been well established.[57] Furthermore, large doses of benzene had been shown to cause chromosomal aberrations in laboratory animals. Doses of 0.2 mg per kg per day, which cause leucopenia, also result in persistent chromatid and chromosome aberrations in the marrow cells in rabbits.[58] Mice and rats are similarly affected.[59] And in cells in vitro, including cultured human cells, high levels of benzene (molar concentrations) cause chromatid breaks and gaps, and appear to act synergistically with the toxic effects of radiation.[60]

Studies of such effects on workers exposed to relatively low levels of benzene, however, showed decidedly mixed results. In 1978 OSHA cited six studies, characterizing three of them as positive and three as negative. One of the studies it considered positive was considered by its authors to be only suggestive. They had reported that nine "seemingly healthy refinery workers exposed to 'low levels' of benzene" did display a significantly elevated incidence of chromosome aberrations relative to controls,[61] but this incidence of aberrations was considered by another investigator to be within "the normal range."[62] In the second such study there appeared to be considerable variation in the responses of exposed workers, with only a few members of the exposed group showing markedly increased rates of chromosome breaks.[63] In contrast, one of the negative studies found no increased incidence of chromosome aberrations among workers who had been "exposed to approximately 12 ppm for an average period of 13 years."[64]

In 1979 Dante Picciano, then at OSHA, reported that workers exposed to benzene—and possibly to other solvents—at levels ranging from 1 to 10 ppm were significantly more likely to display chromosome breaks and marker (abnormally structured) chromosomes than were individuals with no occupational exposure.[65] He also reported the dose-response relationship shown in Table 5.2.

These studies have since been heavily criticized. For one thing, the individuals in the control group tended to be younger than those in the exposed group, and other investigators have suggested that the effects studied may increase with age.[66] Picciano, in response, cited another study in which the frequencies of chromosome breaks did not increase with age.[67] Furthermore, Picciano argued that he found no association between age and chromosome breaks and markers among the workers in the exposed group of his study.

Some critics simply reject Picciano's findings. Reporting on the public comments received in response to its listing of benzene as a hazardous air pollutant, EPA reported: "Although commenters did not disagree with EPA's conclusion that benzene can cause chromosome breakage in humans, they were divided on the exposure levels at which such damage occurs and on the implications of the observed changes. Several commenters asserted that these effects result only from high exposures, in excess of 10 ppm, and that 'no reliable evidence' exists to link subclinical benzene exposure to chromosome

Table 5.2 Benzene exposure and chromosome breaks.

Exposure to benzene	Individuals with lymphocytes who display both breaks and marker chromosomes (percentage)
"None"	3
Up to 1 ppm	21
1–2.5 ppm	25
2.5–10 ppm	33

Source: D. Picciano, "Cytogenetic Study of Workers Exposed to Benzene," Environmental Research, 19 (1979): 33–38.

aberrations."[68] EPA sided with Picciano and cited another, apparently unpublished, study of Dow Chemical workers[69] as evidence that "increased chromosome breakage [was linked] to benzene exposure well below the OSHA standard of 10 ppm time-weighted-average." At the same time EPA found no clinical correlates (that is, no functional changes) associated with the increased incidences of chromosomal changes.

Here, then, is another complexity of the science-policy interface in the regulation of chemical toxins. Not only do we have the usual debates over what effects occurred, but we also encounter disagreements about the significance of certain effects. Given our limited understanding of human biology, we don't always know what might lead to what. Extrapolating from observations of biological effects to policy conclusions of "material impairment" or "incapacitating illness" involves a complex mixture of technical and ethical reasoning.

▪ Cancer in Laboratory Animals

As noted previously, one contrast between benzene and formaldehyde is that animal and human data have played opposite roles in the two cases. Formaldehyde regulation has been driven by laboratory animal test data, and benzene by human case reports and epidemiology.

Until quite recently, benzene and arsenic were considered to be the only two chemicals for which convincing evidence of carcinogenicity existed for humans and not for laboratory animals. As recently as 1982 Goldstein and coworkers wrote: "In man, acute myeloblastic leukemia is . . . clearly associated with benzene exposure . . . there is no evidence that benzene produces myelogenous leukemia in laboratory animals despite more than 5 decades of study using various dosage levels and routes in mice, guinea pigs, rats, and rabbits."[70] This was the case, even though benzene readily induced many other myelotoxic responses in laboratory animals.

Recent results of chronic bioassays from Maltoni's laboratory in Italy and from the National Toxicology Program (NTP) in this country changed the situation markedly. Benzene was shown to be a carcinogen in laboratory animals for organs unrelated to the hematopoeitic system. This raised the possibility that benzene might also pose a carcinogenic risk to different human organs through completely different mechanisms.

Maltoni and coworkers reported the first demonstration of benzene-induced tumors in rats in 1979; their final results were published in 1983.[71] Rats were exposed to liquid benzene via stomach tube and to benzene in air by inhalation. The relevance to human risk of the former experimental exposure route is often questioned, but the inhalation experiments are directly relevant to policy. Inhaled benzene appeared to induce four types of tumors: Zymbal gland tumors, liver tumors (hepatomas), mammary tumors, and lymphoreticular leukemias. The authors of the study concluded: "Benzene is a potent carcinogen, since it not only enhances the incidence of tumors frequently occurring in untreated animals of the tested colony, but also produces infrequent or unusual tumors in the animals used."[72]

Critics, however, have contested the meaning of each of the results for purposes of assessing human risk. Humans have no Zymbal gland or its equivalent. The hepatomas appeared to be only secondary to liver disease, surprisingly induced by benzene. The data on mammary tumors were of borderline statistical significance, and the leukemias were not of a cell type associated with benzene-induced leukemia in humans. James Jandl has noted that Sprague Dawley rats typically have about a 2 percent spontaneous incidence of Zymbal gland tumors, which is not much different from the incidence in Maltoni's benzene-treated rats.[73] Moreover, the experimental exposures were quite high—200 ppm and 300 ppm for four or seven hours per day, five days per week. The authors themselves wrote: "The need for more experimental research is emphasized, particularly to assess the carcinogenic effects of low doses."[74]

Maltoni's observations were later confirmed and extended by the 1983 NTP bioassay of benzene in rats and mice.[75] The NTP study also drew criticism because the animals were exposed to benzene only by stomach tube and only at relatively high doses. Nonetheless, the variety of organs in which tumors arose, and the fact that the incidence of many of the observed tumors increased with dose led the NTP to conclude that there is "clear evidence of carcinogenicity of benzene" in the rats and mice tested. Their data are summarized in Tables 5.3 and 5.4.

Finally, Goldstein and coworkers reported the induction of three cases of myelogenous leukemia among 295 rats and mice inhaling benzene at levels of 100 or 300 ppm. The authors acknowledged that this incidence is not statistically significantly higher ($p = 0.15$) than

Table 5.3 Results of the NTP bioassay of benzene in rats.[a]

Sex	Dose (mg/kg)	Incidence of tumors (percentage)			
		Carcinoma (Zymbal gland)	Squamous cell carcinoma (skin)	Squamous cell papilloma (skin)	Squamous cell carcinoma (oral cavity)
Male	0	4	0	0	2
	50	12	10	4	18
	100	20	6	2	32
	200	34	16	10	38
Female	0	0	—	—	2
	25	10	—	—	10
	50	10	—	—	24
	100	28	—	—	18

Source: National Toxicology Program, *Technical Report on the Toxicology and Carcinogenesis Studies of Benzene in F344/N Rats and B6C3F1 Mice* (Washington, D.C.: Department of Health and Human Services, 1983).

a. Rats were exposed in groups of 50 to benzene in corn oil by stomach tube at the doses listed, 5 days per week, for 103 weeks. Only tumor types that were significantly increased in benzene-treated animals are summarized here.

the zero percent incidence among the control animals in the study, but they wrote: "To the best of our knowledge, myelogenous leukemia has not been recorded in experimentally untreated Sprague-Dawley rats or CD-1 mice . . . [This absence] suggests that the present observations are due to a direct effect of benzene inhalation."[76] Jandl was skeptical. He noted that several inbred strains of rats have high (20–30 percent) rates of spontaneous incidence of myelogenous leukemia and that Sprague Dawley rats are mongrels, thus implying that the three cases observed by Goldstein's group may well have been spontaneous, not induced by benzene.[77]

These data raised the question whether regulators should worry about risks of cancer other than leukemia in humans exposed to benzene. Resolving this issue depends in part upon understanding the mechanisms of benzene toxicity and deciding whether these mechanisms are similar in rodents and in humans. This issue is very important for standard setting because most of the arguments for a threshold in the benzene dose-response function focus on benzene's myelotoxicity. If in addition it is a "classical" carcinogen in man, then the case for making the conventional presumption of a no-threshold, linear dose-response function is strengthened.

Table 5.4 Results of the NTP bioassay of benzene in mice.

Sex	Dose (mg/kg)	Lymphoma	Carcinoma (Zymbal gland)	Adenoma or carcinoma (alveolar bronchiolar)	Adenoma (Harderian gland)	Squamous cell carcinoma (preputial gland)	Benign tumors (ovary)	Carcinoma (mammary gland)	Carcinosarcoma (mammary gland)	Adenoma or carcinoma (hepatocellular)
						Incidence of tumor (percentage)				
Male	0	8	0	20	0	0	—	—	—	—
	25	19	2	33	19	6	—	—	—	—
	50	18	8	38	26	36	—	—	—	—
	100	31	43	43	22	57	—	—	—	—
Female	0	31	0	8	—	—	0	6	0	8
	25	53	0	12	—	—	2	4	0	27
	50	48	2	22	—	—	24	10	2	26
	100	39	6	31	—	—	15	20	8	14

Source: National Toxicology Program, Technical Report on the Toxicology and Carcinogenesis Studies of Benzene in F344/N Rats and B6C3F1 Mice (Washington, D.C.: Department of Health and Human Services, 1983).

a. Mice were exposed in groups of 50 to benzene in corn oil by stomach tube at the doses listed, 5 days per week, for 103 weeks. At least 42 animals were available for observation in each group. The table summarizes incidences only in tumor types which were significantly increased in benzene-treated animals. See source for more details.

• Mechanisms of Toxicity

The pattern of evidence from tests of benzene's toxicity is somewhat surprising. In particular, its genetic toxicology (its effect on chromosomes) is not consistent with the usual pattern. Most chemical carcinogens are mutagens, and most chromosome-damaging agents are mutagens. But benzene is carcinogenic and it damages chromosomes, yet it is not a mutagen, nor are any of its major metabolites. Benzene is definitely negative when tested in the presence or absence of metabolic activation in the Ames assay of mutagenicity.[78] It also fails to mutate *Drosophila* larvae, another classical test.[79]

These anomalies lead some to argue that benzene may be a nonclassical (or, "threshold") carcinogen—that is, its carcinogenicity is secondary to its bone marrow toxicity. Other analysts lean toward the opposite notion, that benzene is a classical carcinogen, especially in light of long-term bioassay results in rats and mice.

There is, of course, no widely agreed-upon answer to the question: "How does benzene cause leukemia?" The mechanisms of action of *all* carcinogens, and the underlying biology of cancer itself, remain largely unknown. There are the beginnings of some understanding, some intriguing clues, and it is exactly in the interpretation and extrapolation of these clues that disagreements arise.

As we noted in our discussion of formaldehyde, most arguments that the mechanisms of carcinogenicity should be considered in regulatory policymaking are, in effect, arguments that there might be a "safe" level of exposure to a carcinogen. The mechanistic speculations suggest that low levels of benzene are less risky than might be projected by using a linear dose-response relationship to extrapolate from the risks attributable to high benzene levels. The implications for standard setting are obvious.

The predominant mechanistic argument is that benzene causes leukemia only through its toxic effects upon the bone marrow. These toxic effects require high and repeated doses, although just how high remains a matter of considerable disagreement. Investigators have not reported marrow dysfunction in workers exposed at or below 10 ppm. A majority of hematologists consider the threshold for benzene-induced myelotoxicity to be well over 10 ppm, so they are generally supportive of current OSHA policy. A minority of those who subscribe to this general outlook nonetheless argue that the current OSHA standard of 10 ppm is too high, on the grounds that it may be too close to the threshold to provide an adequate margin of safety.

Many hematologists (and others) are impressed by the similarity between the effects of benzene and those of several other chemicals known to cause first myelotoxicity and then leukemia. These compounds include the drug chloramphenicol, some alkylating agents used in cancer chemotherapy, and ionizing radiation. All these agents cause dose-dependent myelotoxicity, myelosuppression, and aplasia. The clinical courses for individuals exposed to these agents appear to be quite similar. Some of those who are heavily exposed die within a year as a direct result of the aplasia. Some survive the aplasia, or even appear to recover fully, but succumb to acute myelogenous leukemia within several years. Some recover without further adverse consequences. The transitions from aplasia to leukemia, it is argued, are similar in kind and in frequency for all those agents, although no one understands the reasons for, or mechanisms of, these transitions.

An alternative view is that frank myelotoxicity is not a necessary precursor to benzene-induced leukemia. There are diverse positions here, but each is supportive of a relatively aggressive regulatory response. One position is that myelotoxicity does necessarily precede benzene-induced leukemia, but that the myelotoxicity may be mild, subclinical, and therefore go undetected. The marrow has enough reserve, according to this argument, that some marrow cells can be destroyed with no detectable loss of function. If an agent destroyed 10 percent of the marrow, say, it might lead to only mild cytopenia and allow regeneration to full capacity. But the proliferation involved in that regeneration might pose a risk of cancerous overgrowth—that is, of leukemia.

Alternatively, some assert that the correlation between benzene-induced myelotoxicity and leukemia may not reflect a causal connection. Instead, both may be manifestations of the marrow's response to high levels of benzene exposure. Myelotoxicity appears to precede leukemia only because it is a relatively acute response, from which some individuals recover, while leukemia is a chronic response that is generally fatal. If the mechanisms resulting in the two different diseases are essentially independent, leukemia could arise without being preceded by marrow toxicity.

Various analysts' views about the mechanisms of benzene's toxicity tend to determine their views about the potential effectiveness of medical surveillance of workers as a matter of policy. Jandl, for example, argues that benzene works its effects upon the bone marrow in an unusually, indeed notoriously, slow manner.[80] As marrow function becomes compromised, the blood picture begins to change:

platelet levels drop, circulating lymphocytes diminish in number, and red cells decline in number and may become enlarged. These processes can be monitored by frequent checking and, unless the marrow is almost completely destroyed, might be spontaneously reversed by cessation of exposure to benzene. According to Jandl, bone marrow is remarkably capable of regenerating normal cell numbers and functions, even after some 50 percent of the marrow has been destroyed. For workers exposed to benzene, then, one might have an almost unique opportunity to detect and stop the progression of precarcinogenic states.

Others are less convinced that medical surveillance could be of much benefit to benzene-exposed workers; by the time characteristic abnormalities appear in the blood, it may be too late. Acute myelogenous leukemia, they stress, is a serious and usually fatal disease. There is no guarantee that AML or a precursor state could be detected at an early, reversible stage. Even a diagnosis of aplastic anemia—which proceeds through a series of more easily recognizable and reversible early stages—is not completely straightforward. Irons claims that in laboratory animals leukocyte counts may approach normal ranges, even after 90 percent of the bone marrow cells have been destroyed by benzene.[81] In other words, the marrow could be all but demolished while the white cell count reflected little cause for alarm. In general, the kinetics of lymphocytes in the circulation are so complex that conclusions concerning lymphocyte production cannot be drawn from measurement of blood lymphocyte levels.[82] It is possible to biopsy the marrow directly, but such an onerous procedure would find little acceptance in a program of medical surveillance of exposed workers.

The issue is further complicated because some believe that benzene exposure may induce a variety of human cancers, only some of which can be detected by blood sampling and testing. And, clearly, any chromosomal damage from benzene would be detected by routine blood counts.

In addition to their concern about false negatives in medical surveillance, critics also worry about false positives. They feel that at least some of the markers of benzene-induced marrow toxicity are too variable and/or nonspecific to form the basis of a mandated medical surveillance program. For example, white blood cell levels may be elevated not only by leukemia but also by various infections, smoking, and other factors. And as we noted earlier, the appropriateness of medical surveillance, and the responses attendant upon positive findings, are part of the larger issues of standard-setting policy.

Metabolism

To interpret the evidence from laboratory animals on cancers other than leukemia, it would be helpful to know whether benzene is metabolized similarly in rodents and in humans. For another established human carcinogen, 2-naphthylamine, there are crucial differences in metabolism between the two groups. Rodents lack the enzyme system that transforms the compound into its ultimately carcinogenic form, so they do not develop bladder cancer from it. Humans possess the enzymes and do develop the cancer. Dogs are like humans in this respect and are therefore the animal model used to study 2-naphthylamine-induced bladder cancer. Results from rodents in this case are clearly irrelevant.

Benzene does appear to be sufficiently similarly metabolized in rodents and in humans that the former can serve as a model for the latter. OSHA, for example, stated: "The similarities in the metabolism of benzene and similar effects on bone marrow toxicity in both animals and humans would tend to support the use of rats and mice for bioassay studies on the carcinogenicity of benzene."[83] The two groups cannot be all that similar, of course, since benzene does not seem to cause leukemia in rodents, while it does cause leukemia in humans. The point, though, is that many feel that the solid tumors that arise in rats and mice exposed to benzene cannot be ruled out, at least on the basis of metabolism, as possible responses in humans.

The actual metabolic patterns of benzene are unusually complex and too incompletely understood for information about them to be very useful to the regulatory process. Is this likely to change soon? Are a few more experiments—or even many more experiments—on the metabolism of benzene likely to provide a useful picture?

Some analysts are optimistic. Goldstein, for example, asked, "How can mechanistically oriented studies lead to information pertinent to deciding the regulatory approach to benzene?" He answered that studies might be undertaken "to identify and characterize the as yet unknown metabolite(s) of benzene responsible for hematotoxicity." He states that "toxicokinetic studies of an oncogenic metabolite might reveal whether such a metabolite is formed at any level of benzene or only after other detoxification steps have been exhausted."[84] This is potentially music to the ears of those who oppose tighter regulation of benzene. Imagine that the carcinogenic form of benzene is discovered, but is found not to exist below a certain level of exposure!

Others wonder, whether such a spectacular discovery, if it were made, should alter regulatory approaches. How convincing is it to find "the" carcinogenic metabolite in the absence of a complete understanding of carcinogenesis? Is it even enough to learn what in benzene causes leukemia, or must one also understand the other metabolites that might cause the solid tumors suggested by the animal studies? The answers to these questions involve both time and generalizability. The program of mechanistic research will take years—possibly decades—and the results may vary greatly from carcinogen to carcinogen. Nonetheless, as we discuss in Chapter 7, we believe that mechanistic research offers the best hope of clarifying the magnitude of low-dose cancer risks.

• Conclusions

Our review of the scientific evidence on benzene makes it clear why it has been so difficult to use existing knowledge in standard setting. Some of the difficulty arises—as we described in Chapter 4—from the imprecise and ambiguous language of legislative and judicial pronouncements.

Standard setters want to know dose-response functions, especially at low levels of exposure. Yet the epidemiological data simply cannot be used to answer that question with any precision. Conflicts arise about the interpretation of particular studies, about the persuasiveness of various types of studies, and about the ways information from diverse sources should be combined.

Examples of the first kind of disagreement abound. Should Wong's exposed chemical workers be compared with the low rate in his control group or the higher rate in the general population? Is the overall leukemia rate in Turkey (for comparison with the rate among Aksoy's shoe workers) 6 per 100,000 or 0.66 per 100,000? Did Infante and coworkers know that Pliofilm workers tended to have high rates of leukemia before they began their study, and does that matter? Should the fact that the three leukemia victims in Ott's sample were exposed to low levels of benzene be taken as a signal of benzene's true danger, or does it instead suggest that their diseases were caused by something else?

There are many examples of differences over the credibility of different sources of data. Are clinical case reports valuable, or are they too unreliable and unsystematic for use by regulators? Do results from laboratory animals exposed to benzene via stomach tubes provide biologically important clues, or are they irrelevant exercises? Are mechanistic studies of benzene carcinogenesis the wave of the future and the appropriate basis for regulatory policy, or are they a snare and a delusion designed to slow regulatory action in a world of inevitably imperfect information?

Our review of the scientific evidence suggests that individual scientists do not approach these questions in isolation. They look at each piece of evidence in light of other available data and in terms of their intuitive convictions. Evidence that is suggestive to one is implausible to another exactly because of the way it relates to his or her pattern of beliefs. To be sure, a scientist's broader view of the benzene problem also emerges from, and is influenced by, new experimental and observational data. But the relationship of one to the other is not simple. Data that are persuasive to one may not be compelling to another, in part because of fundamental differences in training and habits of mind.

A scientist's views are, after all, influenced by many factors, including professional training, style of reasoning, and views about wise social policy (which might influence and be influenced by one's place of employment). Furthermore, at least some discussions of apparently narrow issues of study interpretation were apparently influenced by awareness of the strategic implications of such debates for the regulatory process. The closer the discussion comes to policy questions, the clearer and stronger this link became.

Scientists appear to be quite well aware of these and other sources of their own disagreements. They know that personal judgment and intuition play a large role in constructing and interpreting studies. Hence, their opinions of the significance of any given piece of work depend in part on their views of the skill and judgment of the investigators. Sometimes this leads to stereotypical responses— "What do you expect from an industry (or environmental) spokesman?" But it can also reflect a deeper appreciation of the capacities of a particular scientist—"If X found that, it is likely really to be there!"

The problem for regulators is how to extract the best scientific advice from the "experts." What institutions and processes can society create to disentangle all the factors that make up "scientific" results—and to what extent can one even hope to do so?

Before we proceed to that question, we want to look in greater detail at the problems of quantitative risk assessment. For there is increasing pressure on (and from) policy makers to produce such assessments in order to defend and justify decisions.

6 · QUANTIFYING CANCER RISKS

IN THE cases of both benzene and formaldehyde we have seen agencies rely increasingly upon quantitative cancer risk assessments. Since the Supreme Court's 1980 benzene decision, federal agencies have felt compelled to use such numerical risk estimates to support both priority-setting and standard-setting decisions. So far we have reported numerical risk estimates without much comment about how they are calculated, how well they are supported by scientific evidence, and what their uncertainties are. In this chapter these questions are explored in some detail.

For toxins other than carcinogens, federal agencies for decades have made decisions without doing quantitative risk assessments. Instead, data from acute and chronic animal bioassays have been used to establish a no-observable-effect level, which is then divided by a "safety factor" to establish a "safe" or permissible exposure level for humans. A safety factor of 100 has been traditional: a factor of 10 to allow for the possibility that humans are an order of magnitude more sensitive than the test species, and another factor of 10 to cover variation among test species.

Some observers have suggested that the same approach be used for carcinogens. For example, one analyst proposes the use of a safety factor of 5,000. This would include, along with the two factors of 10, another factor of 10 for carcinogenesis "on the theory that this type of action may be less reversible than some others," and a factor of 5 because the NOEL in even a large and well-designed bioassay may be five times greater than the "true" no-effects level for a particular tumor type in a particular species exposed to a particular chemical.[1]

The traditional toxicological approach could be applied to formaldehyde and benzene. For formaldehyde the NOEL for rats in the CIIT

This chapter was written with the assistance of Scott Wolff.

bioassay was 2 ppm. This exposure level is already lower than the OSHA standard before being divided by a safety factor. The commonly applied safety factor of 100 would posit the permissible level of human exposure to formaldehyde at 0.02 ppm. For benzene the NOEL in animals varies from species to species but is never lower than 100 ppm. That would imply a safe level of 100/100 = 1 ppm. In principle, the same method could be used for human data with an adjustment in the safety factor. For example, if benzene is not observed to cause leukemia in humans at 100 ppm, then a safety factor of 10 (to account, say, for variations in human susceptibility) would lead to a permissible exposure level of 10 ppm. A key problem, of course, is that the levels of exposure to benzene that were associated with excess leukemia in the past are not known with any precision.

Some analysts prefer the use of NOELs and safety factors because, they argue, the attempt to quantify cancer risks is premature. Something as unsophisticated and arbitrary as a safety factor, they contend, mirrors our current lack of sophistication in understanding the mechanisms of carcinogenesis. And reliance on the NOEL places emphasis on the experimental dose closest to the generally smaller human doses.

It is fair to say, however, that this traditional toxicological approach has been largely rejected by federal regulatory agencies for use with carcinogens.[2] One reason is that some theories of carcinogenesis imply that any exposure to a carcinogen, however small, will increase a person's risk of contracting cancer. This implies that there is no no-effects level. Others object to reliance on NOELs because they fear that manufacturers planning to produce a chemical would have it tested in fewer rather than more animals. The smaller the number of animals, the more likely it is that a small effect will appear to be no effect. And others have noted that safety factors are arbitrary, while quantitative risk assessment offers promise of being more "scientific."[3]

As this chapter shows, quantitative risk assessments have not proven to be the panacea that they were intended to be. Agency risk estimates convey both too much and too little confidence in science. The estimates convey overconfidence in the sense that the true extent of biological uncertainty and scientific conflict is not reflected in the published numbers. At the same time, the procedures used by agency analysts often do not incorporate all of the relevant biological information and the final numbers often fly in the face of technical intuition and judgment. To better understand the nature of these difficulties, it is useful to explore the major analytical decisions in risk assessment and the procedures currently employed by federal agencies.

• The Essential Problem

The difficulties of doing quantitative risk assessment arise from the lack of information about human dose-response curves at the doses that are important to regulatory policy. For a variety of reasons, the low-dose region of the human dose-response curve for cancer is generally unobservable. Epidemiologists often must work with inadequate data. The human data that are available typically involve historic exposures that are both poorly documented and generally much higher than those of current regulatory concern. Similarly, we have little data from laboratory animal bioassays at the dose levels of regulatory interest. Questions also arise about how the animal data should be interpreted and the extent to which humans resemble the test species.

Whether the risk analyst is trying to extrapolate from high to low doses, from mouse to man, or both, the challenge is to use the known to predict the unknown (or at least the observed to forecast the unobserved). If all chemicals caused cancer through the same biological mechanisms, we might be able to accumulate enough knowledge of the process to model a particular case with relatively little data. For example, if the physiologic and metabolic differences between animals and humans were the same for all substances, then we could apply the same interspecies "correction factor" to each chemical.

The world is not this simple. Our cases suggest that the processes by which chemical exposures produce cancer vary widely. Benzene does not act like formaldehyde; leukemia is not like squamous cell nasal carcinoma. There are often significant differences in the way particular compounds affect different species. Rats don't contract leukemia from breathing benzene; humans do. Rats get nasal carcinomas from formaldehyde, but people may not. Hence, no single interspecies extrapolation rule will be accurate (or even equally conservative) in all cases.

Since cancer risks are always assessed in the face of such great uncertainty, disagreements arise about how to proceed. Indeed, it is likely that no responsible scientist would even try to make (or take much interest in) such numerical estimates were it not for the pressure to do so for policy reasons. As a result, the boundary between science and policy runs through many of the methodological disputes about cancer risk assessment. In the heat of particular controversies, the disputants often fail (even after much effort) to distinguish among the grounds for their arguments. Methods are sometimes defended on the grounds that they are "scientific" and at other times on the grounds that they are "conservative." Confusion is rampant, as we shall see.

As a context for what follows, it is worth noting that there is a conceptual framework that purports to tell us how such problems should be handled. That framework is a branch of applied mathematics called "decision theory."[4] It offers two main principles. First, risk assessors should make a conscious and self-critical attempt to distinguish between estimates of the extent of cancer risk and values concerning how much effort society should devote to reducing various levels of risk. Having made this distinction, the risk assessor should then try to quantify explicitly the magnitude of uncertainty about his or her estimates of cancer risks. A single, or "point," estimate is not sufficiently informative. The full extent of uncertainty—biological and statistical—must be characterized quantitatively. Making specific estimates of the probabilities of various outcomes can help the regulator think about the extent of potential gains from acquiring better information about the chemical. In addition, the regulator should try to quantify explicitly both how "risk averse" (or conservative) he or she wants to be by quantifying just how unacceptable various rates of cancer would be relative to each other and to other kinds of policy outcomes. Thus, the decision analyst urges regulators to quantify *separately* the likelihood of various health outcomes and their degree of happiness or unhappiness if the various outcomes were to occur.[5]

One striking feature of the review we are about to provide is how thoroughly such decision-theoretical ideas are ignored by cancer risk assessors. In part the problem is with decision theory, which does not yet offer a clear program for obtaining all of the necessary quantification. But part of the problem lies with risk assessors in federal agencies, where there are institutional incentives to conceal uncertainty and neglect scientific evidence and judgments that run counter to prevailing guidelines. It is therefore useful to describe how quantitative cancer risk assessment is currently practiced by federal agencies.

• Extrapolating from High to Low Doses

The task of extrapolating from high to low doses arises with both animal and human data. Standard practice is to "fit" some sort of mathematical function to the observed dose-response data and use that function to project responses into the low-dose region, where actual responses have not been observed. This requires two main choices: what mathematical model to fit and what statistical method to use when fitting it.

Low-Dose Extrapolation of Animal Data

At least half a dozen tractable mathematical models can be used with experimental bioassay data.[6] Generally they all fit such data fairly well and have some bases in cancer biology. It is apparent, though, that the models often predict quite different carcinogenic responses at doses below the experimental range. Some of these models are described in Table 6.1.

Although there is considerable uncertainty about which model best reflects the biology of any particular chemical carcinogen, the multistage model is by far the most widely used in the federal government. All three major federal agencies—CPSC, EPA, and OSHA—used it in their formaldehyde deliberations. It was also used by EPA, OSHA, and the California Department of Health Services to assess the recent bioassay data on benzene. The multistage model is an exponential model of the following form:

$$P = 1 - exp[-(q_0 + q_1d + q_2d^2 + \ldots + q_nd^n)].$$

Doing some algebra and then taking the natural logarithm of both sides yields:

$$\ln(1 - P) = q_0 + q_1d + q_2d^2 + \ldots + q_nd^n,$$

where P is the probability of developing cancer after lifetime exposure to dose d of a chemical and the q's are coefficients estimated from the dose-response data.[7] The underlying biological theory is that a developing tumor progresses through several different stages before it becomes clinically detectable, and each stage of the process can be influenced by exposure to carcinogens.[8]

It is a flexible model in that it can take different forms—in response to different data sets—by assuming a different number of dose-related stages. Each power of dose in the above equation corresponds

Table 6.1 Mathematical models for low-dose extrapolation of animal bioassay data.

Tolerance distribution models

Assume that each member of a population has a threshold or tolerance level below which that individual will not develop cancer in response to the chemical exposure in question.

Assume that variability among individual threshold levels can be described in terms of a probability distribution.

The probit, logit, and Weibull models can be generated by adopting different probability distributions to describe individual variations in tolerance.

Mechanistic models

Assume that low-dose extrapolation can be based on a mechanistic theory of carcinogenesis.

Assume that a tumor originates from a single cell that has been damaged by either a chemical or one of its metabolites.

Examples include the one-hit, multihit, and multistage models.

Time-to-tumor models

Presume that the complex relationship among dose, tumor latency, and cancer risk can be modeled.

Examples include the Armitage-Doll, Hartley-Sielken, Weibull distribution, and log normal distribution models.

Sources: U.S. Office of Science and Technology Policy, "Chemical Carcinogens: A Review of the Science and Its Associated Principles," *Federal Register*, 50 (1985): 10438–10439; and Paolo F. Ricci and Lawrence S. Molton, "Regulating Cancer Risk," *Environmental Science and Technology*, 19, no. 6 (1985): 473–479.

to a stage. When the model was originally designed, the number of stages was assumed to be no greater than one less than the number of dose levels in the experiment that generates the dose-response data.

Once a mathematical form is selected for low-dose extrapolation, a statistical technique must be selected to estimate the model's coefficients. Least squares regression, a common statistical method, is generally not helpful because of the nonlinear forms of the model and the small number of experimental data points. The standard practice among risk assessors is to use the "maximum likelihood" technique, which determines—for a given model and assumed random error component—what coefficient estimates make it most likely that the observed experimental data would be generated.

To provide some measure of statistical uncertainty, risk assessors often generate confidence intervals around the maximum likelihood estimates, or MLEs. A 90 to 95 percent upper confidence limit (UCL) is commonly reported, although there is no particular reason—other than that they are "round numbers"—for choosing these particular limits. The confidence limits, also called upper bounds, capture only the random errors, given the model. They do not convey any uncertainty about whether the model was properly specified or whether the model selected was the correct one. They therefore understate the overall degree of uncertainty.

Formaldehyde. Suppose, for the sake of argument, that we are willing to accept multistage as the appropriate model and maximum likelihood as the appropriate estimation technique. What risk estimates for formaldehyde are generated based on the CIIT rat data? Table 6.2 provides two sets of estimates based on subtly different analytical choices, which lead to some significant differences in risk estimates. For example, OSHA's MLEs are consistently one to two orders of magnitude smaller than those reported by Clement Associates, a private consulting firm. The UCLs, though, vary by a factor of only about two.

The major reason for the disparate estimates is the number of stages assumed in the two analyses. Clement used a version of the multistage equation in which only d^3 was multiplied by a nonzero coefficient (q_3).[9] OSHA used dose to the fourth and fifth powers, which yields a fitted dose-response function that is more nonlinear. Since the fitted curve can now come closer to the small observed

Table 6.2 Formaldehyde risk estimates based on the multistage model.

Exposure level (ppm)	Excess lifetime cancers per 100,000 exposed workers			
	OSHA		Clement	
	MLE	UCL	MLE	UCL
3	71	834	620	930
1	0.6	264	23	130
0.5	0.03	132	2.8	58
0.1	0.001	26	<0.1	11

Source: Occupational Safety and Health Administration, "Occupational Exposure to Formaldehyde," *Federal Register*, 50 (1985): 50458, 50460.

response at 5.6 ppm, it also tends to predict smaller risks at low doses.

Proponents of a fifth-degree polynomial argue that the fourth and fifth powers of dose are necessary to capture the extreme nonlinearity in the data points from the CIIT rat study. In short, five stages fit the experimental data better than do three stages.[10] Advocates of three stages respond that the multistage model was not designed to allow more stages than the number of experimental dose levels. (What matters statistically is the number of terms relative to the number of data points—that is, the degrees of freedom available—and not the size of the exponent on the largest term.) They argue also that the fit is not "much" better and that there is no biological reason to prefer five stages to three.[11]

The choice of a mathematical model can also exert a powerful influence on the resulting risk estimates. Table 6.3 presents a comparison of risk estimates from five models. (Note that the multistage estimates presented here—this time based on a three-stage polynomial but with a different treatment of the sacrificed animals in the CIIT experiment—offer yet another set of numbers.) As we might expect, the differences in the risk estimates that result from using the various models are quite large. It should be emphasized, however, that these sensitivities to model selection in the case of formaldehyde are "small" relative to those for extrapolations of data on many other chemicals. This is because occupational exposures to formaldehyde are much closer to the bioassay doses than is often the case. The greater the difference between actual doses and bioassay doses, the more opportunity there is for the various models to diverge in their low-dose risk estimates.

Federal agencies have developed a strong commitment to the multistage model, but the reasons for this preference are not entirely clear.[12] It is also apparent that EPA and CPSC (but not OSHA) have decided to rely on the 95 percent upper confidence limits instead of the MLEs.[13] Here the mixing of policy and science comes to the forefront. Agencies want to be sure not to underestimate cancer risk. So rather than relying on MLEs or some overall "best guess" of risk, they intentionally aim high in order to be conservative. And instead of always calling the upper limit an upper limit, agencies sometimes call it an "estimate" from the linearized multistage model. This terminology is based on the observation that the 95 percent upper limit of risk from the multistage model tends to be a linear function of dose at sufficiently low doses, even though the MLE may behave in a non-

Table 6.3 Formaldehyde risk estimates for rats based on alternative mathematical models.

Exposure level (ppm)	Excess lifetime cancers per 100,000									
	Multistage		Probit		Logit		Weibull		Multihit	
	MLE	UCL	MLE	UCL	MLE	UCL	MLE	UCL	MLE	UCL
3	43.4	633	23.9	264	59.9	315	81.5	329	0.8	212
1	7.4	411	3.8	73	16.2	138	27.2	161	0.4	23
0.5	0.4	204	0.4	12	2.9	40	6.5	56	0	0.2
0.1	0	102	0.1	3	0.8	15	2.2	23	0	0

Source: Kenneth G. Brown, "Risk Assessment of Laboratory Rats and Mice Chronically Exposed to Formaldehyde Vapors," Risk Analysis, 5(1985):171; reprinted in Federal Register, 50 (1985): 50460.

linear fashion over all doses. EPA frequently emphasizes that the linearized multistage model is conservative and provides a "plausible upper limit" on actual risk.

When criticized for mixing science and policy, EPA responds that low-dose linearity is scientifically the most plausible hypothesis.[14] Since humans are exposed to a large background of carcinogenic exposure, low doses of any particular carcinogen may add to the overall load. This may produce a linear segment of the dose-response curve for each carcinogen. One advocate of this view, statistician Kenneth Crump, has stated, concerning formaldehyde, that "I hold to the view that the true response is probably linear at low doses . . . we can't rule out the possibility that the risks are about as large as those predicted by the linearized multistage model."[15]

An alternative view, held by statistician Robert Sielken, is that the linearized multistage model produces upper bounds on risk, not estimates of risk. He argues further that the computer programs used by federal agencies, such as GLOBAL 79, do not produce normal upper confidence limits (numbers based solely on variability in the fitting technique). Instead the procedures used to generate upper confidence limits are designed to "force" the maximum amount of linearity into the multistage model without creating a very poor fit to the data. In the case of formaldehyde, he argues that the dose-response function is very likely to be nonlinear at low doses—thus arguing against giving credence to the 95 percent upper limit.[16]

The disparity between the MLE and the upper limit is not a trivial matter, because federal agencies often use numerical thresholds in priority setting to help identify significant cancer risks. (For regulators and courts, significance means importance, not "statistical significance.") OSHA has adopted a cutoff of 10^{-3} as a result of the Supreme Court's benzene decision. EPA uses cutoffs ranging from 10^{-3} to 10^{-6}, depending upon the program. It turns out that formaldehyde exposures of 3 ppm constitute a significant risk at OSHA when the UCL is used as the measure. As tables 6.2 and 6.3 show, as levels of exposure to formaldehyde fall, the maximum likelihood estimates of risk vanish to insignificance much more quickly than do the upper confidence levels.

The issue of which number to rely on—the MLE or the UCL—was quite salient in both CPSC's decision about urea-formaldehyde insulation and EPA's formaldehyde decision under the Toxic Substances Control Act. As we saw in Chapter 2, CPSC attempted to regulate on the basis of the UCL of the multistage model, even though the MLE of risk from UFFI was virtually zero. At EPA risk analysts reported that the UCLs of the multistage model suggested that ambient exposure to formaldehyde would cause more than 10,000 excess cancers annually nationwide. The corresponding MLE of risk was about 50 excess cancers nationwide.[17] Although it is EPA's announced policy to rely on the UCLs of the multistage model, the agency did not take any rulemaking action to reduce concentrations of formaldehyde in the ambient air. It may be that regulators are willing to endorse linear, no-threshold models as a matter of general principle, but are also prepared to believe (at least implicitly) in nonlinearities or no-effect thresholds—either of which can imply vanishingly small risks at some doses—if the doses are small enough.

Benzene. As discussed in Chapter 5, benzene is considered a known human leukemogen. Although scientists have not yet succeeded in producing leukemia in animals via benzene exposure, the chemical has been shown to produce other types of cancers in animals. These findings raise the possibility that benzene exposure may cause several forms of cancer in humans. If these risks are to be estimated, we must extrapolate responses involving relatively high exposures in laboratory animal bioassays to lower human exposures.

To reinforce the earlier point about the importance of the choice of mathematical model (shape of the dose-response function), we examine some estimates of human cancer risk based on extrapolation of results from Maltoni's bioassay (see Chapter 5). The resulting risk estimates for continuous occupational exposure to 1 ppm benzene are summarized in Table 6.4. In this case the three models yield roughly

Table 6.4 Benzene risk estimates based on Maltoni's 1982 animal bioassay.

Model	Excess cancers per 1,000 workers at 1 ppm
Multistage	
MLE	3
UCL	34
Probit	
MLE	3
UCL	70
Weibull	
MLE	10
UCL	80

Source: "Preliminary Results of EPA's Carcinogen Assessment Group," *Federal Register,* 50 (1985): 50537–50538.

comparable MLEs at the 1 ppm level. Note, however, that the linearized multistage or UCL does *not* produce the highest estimate of risk in this case. The UCLs for both the probit and Weibull forms are even larger. Apparently the shape parameter for the Weibull model was estimated to be less than 1 for this data set, which means that the estimated dose-response curve is actually concave downward ("supralinear") at low doses.[18] This result underscores the limits of the claim that the linearized multistage model will always provide an upper limit on actual risk.

Low-Dose Extrapolation of Human Data

When epidemiological data are available, the assessor must again face the same two choices: a mathematical model and a statistical estimation technique. Many mathematical models are biologically plausible, but we found only one that was actually used to generate risk estimates. The so-called one-hit model is of the form:

$$P_d = [1 - e^{(-Bd)}] (1 - P_0),$$

where P_d is excess cancer risk attributable to dose d, P_0 is the relevant background rate of cancer risk, and B is a "potency" coefficient to be estimated from the epidemiological data. In particular, B is sometimes expressed as follows:

$$B = -\ln\{[1 - (SMR/100)P_0]/[1 - P_0]\}/d$$

The risk assessor need "only" obtain historical dose and the standardized mortality ratio (SMR) from an epidemiological study in order to estimate this model. If more than one dose-response point is available, the maximum likelihood method can be used to generate estimates and confidence limits.

The one-hit model, which is a special case of the multistage model, presumes that a single molecule of a carcinogen can alter a cell's DNA in a way that subsequently leads to the development of cancer.[19] It is a no-threshold model: every addition to dose is accompanied by some incremental risk of cancer. It is also a "relative risk" model since it presumes that cancer risk responds to each unit of dose in some constant multiplicative fashion relative to the background rate of cancer. In contrast, an "absolute risk" model, where chemical exposures simply add to the background rate of cancer, is rarely used in quantitative risk assessment, even though it is not biologically implausible.[20]

For formaldehyde, the human data on cancer risk are not of sufficient quality to estimate a dose-response function. For benzene,
though, numerous investigators have used the one-hit model to make
low-dose extrapolations of cancer risk. The pioneer in this effort,
Harvard physicist Richard Wilson, offered a crude "back-of-the-
envelope" calculation at OSHA's 1977 benzene hearings.[21] He projected that workers continuously exposed at the prevailing PEL of 10
ppm would have an annual excess risk of death of 3.5×10^{-5}. He
found that this risk was about the same as that encountered in manufacturing in general and less than that associated with mining, steel
working, fire fighting, or piloting a plane.

Several other risk estimates for benzene have been based on the
one-hit model. The results are summarized as lifetime risk estimates
in Table 6.5. These results are perhaps more alike than one might
have expected, given the scientific conflicts surveyed in Chapter 5.
This convergence reflects the common assumptions and the relatively
small amount of human data on which the numbers are based rather
than the precise state of the "science" of risk assessment.

Because of the poor quality of the underlying data (see Chapter 5)
and the very small number of cases on which the estimates are based,
not everyone is enthusiastic about the exercise. Brian MacMahon, a
prominent epidemiologist at Harvard, writes: "In my view it is ludi-
crous to attempt quantitative risk assessments for benzene at this time
[April 1983]. In one of the sources of data used [Rinsky et al.] estimates of exposure are no better than guesses; in the other [Ott et al.]
the estimate of leukemia is based on the occurrence of only three
cases. No amount of modeling can paper over these basic defects . . .
the presentation of the dressed-up guesses at this time serves no
useful purpose."[22]

Others are a bit more adventurous. An IARC committee commented: "The Working Group found that quantitative estimation of
the human cancer risk which is associated with ·exposure . . . to
benzene was more feasible than seemed initially to be the case. The
Group was impressed that rather large amounts of quantitative information could be extracted from the published epidemiological
studies and that reasonable risk estimations could then be based on
that information."[23]

This same IARC group, however, shied away from the aspects of
quantification related to policy. They estimated the number of excess
cases of leukemia ascribable to 100 ppm benzene, but declined to
extrapolate the risk estimates to levels of exposure near the OSHA

Table 6.5 Benzene risk estimates based on epidemiological data.

Assessors[a]	Cases of leukemia per 1,000 person lifetimes per ppm benzene
Wilson	1
IARC	[b]
Lamm	2.2
Crump and Allen	2–9.5
White, Infante, and Chu	5–16
Luken and Miller	17
California Department of Health Services	22
Carcinogen Assessment Group	24
Hattis and Mendez	26

a. Richard Wilson, Testimony before OSHA on benzene proposal, 1977, mimeo; International Agency for Research on Cancer, *Monographs on the Evaluation of Carcinogenic Risk of Chemicals to Humans,* vol. 29 (Geneva: WHO, 1982); S. Lamm, "Analysis of the Quantitative Assessment of the Leukemogenic Risk from Ambient Exposure to Benzene," Consultants in Epidemiology and Occupational Health, Feb. 1, 1982; K. Crump and B. Allen, "Quantitative Estimates of Risk of Leukemia from Occupational Exposures to Benzene," Report to OSHA, May 1984; M. White, P. Infante, and K. Chu, "A Quantitative Estimate of Leukemia Mortality Associated with Occupational Exposure to Benzene," *Risk Analysis,* 2 (1982): 195–203; Ralph Luken and Stephen G. Miller, "The Benefits and Costs of Regulating Benzene," *Journal of the Air Pollution Control Association,* 31 (Dec. 1981): 1254–1259; California Department of Health Services, *Report to the Scientific Review Panel on Benzene,* Nov. 27, 1984; Carcinogen Assessment Group, *Population Risk to Ambient Benzene Exposure* (Washington, D.C.: Environmental Protection Agency, 1979); D. Hattis and W. Mendez, "Discussion and Critique of the Carcinogen Assessment Group's Report on Population Risk due to Atmospheric Benzene Exposure" (Cambridge, Mass.: MIT Center for Policy Alternatives, May 1980).

b. IARC estimates some 140 to 170 excess cases of leukemia per 1,000 people occupationally exposed to 100 ppm benzene. The linear extrapolation, which IARC did not make, would posit the risk at 1.4 to 1.7 excess leukemias per ppm benzene.

standard of 10 ppm. (In fact, a draft copy of the IARC group's report did contain a risk estimate at 10 ppm, but it was removed by the organization's director because "the data were inadequate to support the estimate.")[24]

Having noted the convergence of the estimates, we must also consider why they diverge at all. Why don't all of the assessors who use the one-hit model report identical results? In part the differences reflect the choice of studies from which to calculate an SMR. It also turns out that the determination of a background rate (P_0) of leukemia is far from straightforward. For example, the major difference between the estimates reported by Richard Wilson and by EPA's Carcinogen Assessment Group (CAG) turns out to derive from different estimates of the background incidence of leukemia in Turkey.

In his early papers Aksoy stated that the annual leukemia incidence in the general Turkish population was 6.0 cases per 100,000.[25] Wilson took him at his word. CAG did not. CAG made three revisions in the estimate and wound up with a background leukemia incidence of 0.66 per 100,000—ten times lower than the figure Aksoy reported and Wilson used.[26]

CAG noted, first, that Aksoy had testified before OSHA in 1977 that the Turkish leukemia rate was 2.5 to 3.0 per 100,000—not 6.0 per 100,000. This rate was for all types of leukemia—myelogenous and lymphocytic. CAG used the lower rate (2.5) as a starting point. Second, CAG argued that only the incidence of myelogenous leukemias should be used as a reference, for it is in those types that benzene has been most strongly implicated. Although there does not seem to be much data on the incidence of these specific types in Turkey, CAG noted that Aksoy found—based on a nonrandom sample of fifty leukemia cases with no known history of benzene exposure—that about half were myelogenous. So CAG divided its lower background rate for all leukemias in half again to arrive at a general incidence of about 1.3 per 100,000.

Third, CAG argued that this figure was still too high because it was not (apparently) adjusted for age. Aksoy's benzene-exposed patients were relatively young, on average in their mid-thirties, when they incurred leukemia. The correct comparison, CAG contended, would be with the background incidence of leukemia among all people in their mid-thirties, not among people of all ages. The average rate for all ages is higher than that for mid-thirty-year-olds because leukemia tends to strike in later years. So CAG divided the background rate in half again, to arrive at a final background rate of 0.66 per 100,000.

Who is right, Wilson or CAG? Is the relative risk for leukemia among Aksoy's shoe workers 13/6 = 2.2 or is it 13/0.66 = 20? Both sides appear to see some merits in the other's approach, judging by the closer convergence of their recent assessments. Wilson now thinks the correct relative risk is about 5 or 6, not 2.[27] CAG has done some recalculating as well, and now posits the relative risk at around 18.[28] Wilson thinks the two approaches are even closer than that: he feels that CAG must have made a simple arithmetic error, because when he used all their assumptions he computed a relative risk of only 13.[29]

Another risk assessment of benzene at low doses, by White, Infante, and Chu, has attracted considerable controversy, even though its estimates are by no means extreme.[30] One reason is that the estimates are based in part on Infante's controversial data on Pliofilm workers. This has rekindled the controversy, reviewed in Chapter 5, over whether Infante's study had accurate exposure data and whether the cluster of seven leukemias was known in advance and, if so, whether SMRs computed from a known cluster are relevant to risk assessment. The risk estimate by White, Infante, and Chu is also based on the study by Ott and coworkers, in which three leukemia deaths were observed among Dow workers exposed to benzene (relative to 0.8 expected). Thus the entire assessment is based on ten cases of leukemia. Some, like MacMahon, consider this number of cases to be too small to support any meaningful inferences—let alone low-dose extrapolations.

Another controversy has arisen over whether White, Infante, and Chu selected modes of analysis that inflated the risk estimates. The disagreement is as follows. If we calculate a relative risk for the leukemias observed among all of the Pliofilm workers, we divide 7 observed cases by 1.25 expected cases, producing a relative risk of 5.6. If instead we calculate a relative risk only for those workers with more than five years of exposure to benzene, we divide 5 cases by 0.23 expected, yielding a relative risk of 21. White, Infante, and Chu used 21, which epidemiologist Philip Cole considers inappropriate.[31] He is especially critical of the exclusion from the risk estimation of workers exposed to benzene for less than five years, followed by the use of those results to predict the risk for workers with less than five years of benzene exposure.

The most heated disputes about low-dose extrapolation of human data tend to occur when the extrapolation spans several orders of magnitude in dose. In those cases the differences in the models and methods have the greatest impact on the results. The estimates of risk from environmental benzene exposures made by EPA and the California Department of Health Services (DHS) raise precisely this question.[32] The exposures of interest to policy makers—exposures in the ambient air—fall in the range of ppb, perhaps five orders of magnitude below the levels demonstrated to be leukemogenic in epidemiological studies. The California DHS argued that benzene should be treated as a substance without a carcinogenic threshold in humans because "no positive evidence exists for this position with respect to benzene."[33] (EPA too has assumed no threshold in several other rulemakings and in the agency's generic carcinogen assessment guidelines.)[34] Using the one-hit model, DHS then projected that the average benzene concentration, 4.6 ppb, in the South Coast Air Basin of Los Angeles would produce 101 excess cases of leukemia per year per 1,000,000 persons.[35] Their projection based on recent animal data was even larger, by a factor of 8. While stressing that these estimates are upper bounds on actual risk, DHS asserts that it is appropriate to be conservative when estimating cancer risk.

A decision theorist would be sympathetic with concerns that any single estimate of risk might be too low. But he or she would be very unsympathetic with the methods used by risk assessors to avoid underestimating risk. An upper bound based on possible random processes within the estimates generated by a single specific model does not tell us how likely it is that the true risk is above or below the reported upper bound because of misspecified modeling, and it says nothing about what our overall best estimate of risk is. This same problem of using uniform rules to calculate conservative risk estimates arises again and again, not just in low-dose extrapolation but also in extrapolations from laboratory animals to humans.

▪ Interspecies Extrapolation

Given the length of latency periods and the limited power of epidemiology to detect human risks, regulators generally cannot wait until they have positive evidence of health effects in people. That would entail too great a risk of failing to regulate some truly harmful substances. The question thus becomes how to utilize alternative data, namely data from laboratory animal bioassays, to predict human cancer risk.

Our cases have called attention to the following general issues in interspecies extrapolation:

▪ If bioassay data are available on more than one strain of a nonhuman species or on more than one nonhuman species, which data should be used for human risk estimation?

▪ How should data on different types of tumors, especially benign versus malignant tumors, be incorporated into human risk estimates?

▪ When responses in a test species are observed at multiple sites or target organs, which responses should be used for estimating human risk?

▪ How should doses administered to animals be converted to equivalent doses for humans?

- How should suspected variations in susceptibility to cancer risk among humans and test animals be incorporated into human risk estimates?

Answering these questions involves a mixture of technical and policy considerations in the face of great uncertainty, and no definitive answers have emerged. Agencies have tried to devise and rely on generic (and rather arbitrary) guidelines to help them decide what to do in specific cases. Yet estimates based on these guidelines are often ignored when they lead to results that are "implausible."

Formaldehyde. In the case of formaldehyde, the tumor site and species used for extrapolation to human risk was dictated largely by the data. Nasal carcinomas are the only confirmed carcinogenic response to formaldehyde in test animals. They occur in both rats and mice, but the results for mice occur only at the highest exposure level. The CIIT investigators believe that rats are more sensitive than mice primarily because mice alter their breathing patterns in response to formaldehyde. The implication is that rats and mice do have comparable responses, if one calculates effective, as opposed to administered, doses to nasal tissues in the two species.

But what does this suggest about potential human risk? Do humans also alter their breathing patterns when exposed to formaldehyde or do they behave more like rats? OSHA's stated view is that "an employee performing a job would generally be unable to lower his or her breathing rate." The rat data are thus "preferred over the results for mice" because "they may represent a situation more typical of human exposure."[36] At very low doses, when formaldehyde cannot be detected by smell or felt by irritation, this assumption seems particularly reasonable.

What about the broader issue of human susceptibility to formaldehyde? Some analysts contend that humans are not obligate nose breathers, which may mean that the effective dose to nasal tissues is lower. Others point out that rats "have approximately twice the relative [nasal] surface area [of] man for filtering inspired air," indicating that "man would receive a smaller target dose than rodents if both were exposed to a similar concentration."[37] Hence, some speculate that humans are less sensitive than rats in this respect.

An alternative view is that humans are presumably more heterogeneous in susceptibility to cancer than any specific strain of rat and are also exposed to many more carcinogenic insults on a daily basis. These considerations lead some observers to speculate that "proportionately more humans (than rats) should develop cancer [from form-aldehyde] at lower doses."[38] On this question the Consensus Workshop on Formaldehyde said only: "Although there are differences in formaldehyde carcinogenicity among different species, at present there is no reason to assume that humans would be more or less susceptible than the rat."[39] OSHA, EPA, and CPSC made the same assumption.

An even more controversial issue is the treatment of the benign tumors (polypoid adenomas) in the CIIT rat study. Federal regulatory guidelines generally call for including benign tumors in quantitative risk assessments.[40] But many scientists argue that formaldehyde should be an exception. As explained in Chapter 3, the polypoid adenomas observed in the exposed rats did not exhibit a positive dose-response relationship. Although polypoid adenomas in general progress to malignant adenocarcinomas, the rate at which they do so in both rats and humans appears to be "very low."[41] And papillomas, the benign counterparts of squamous cell carcinomas, were not observed in the CIIT rat study, although they did appear in the NYU study.

Others argue that the polypoid adenomas should be included. One analyst believes that a malignant neoplasm found in one rat in the CIIT's high-dose group exhibits "similar morphologic features to many of the polypoid adenomas," indicating that "it may represent the malignant counterpart of the polypoid adenoma."[42] Another observer counted two adenocarcinomas in the high-dose group. As shown in Chapter 3, the largest number of polypoid adenomas appeared among rats exposed to 2 ppm formaldehyde. Both EPA and OSHA estimated human cancer risk based on the polypoid adenoma results at 2 ppm. The responses at higher doses were omitted, and a simple linear model was used to extrapolate risk from 2 ppm down to zero dose. The resulting estimates were 1,911 excess cancers per 100,000 workers at 1 ppm, with a 95 percent upper confidence limit of 3,260 per 100,000.

In defense of this approach, OSHA argues that "changes occurring in the nasal passages, leading to squamous cell carcinomas, could have masked the appearance of adenomas at higher doses." EPA speculates that the "cell type needed for these tumors [polypoid adenomas] to occur is lost sooner and to a greater extent with increasing dose." Hence they argue for excluding higher dose data.

CIIT scientists, among others, criticized the omission of the benign responses at 5.6 ppm. At this dose, at which only two small nasal carcinomas were observed, it is unlikely that any polypoid adenomas were "suppressed."[43] Moreover, critics insist that the adenomas occur at a different site within the nasal cavity than do the squamous cell carcinomas. Still others note that CIIT's finding of formaldehyde-produced adenomas in rodents has not yet been replicated, and in any event, most cases of polypoid adenoma in humans are not fatal. The Consensus Workshop on Formaldehyde concluded that "because of different cell types of origin, any evaluation of adenomas [should] be done separately from squamous cell carcinomas."[44]

The line here between scientific and policy judgment is quite blurred. It is conservative to combine the two types of tumors, but this approach may grossly inflate the actual human cancer risk. To ignore the benign tumor data is to run the risk of underestimating actual human risk. If risk estimates are reported separately for the two tumor types, the regulator is left in a quandry about what to make of the disparate estimates. It may make little sense to perform low-dose extrapolation at all for such an apparently odd-shaped dose-response curve—whose shape may be odd because the data are "noisy" and have little biological meaning. Laboratory scientists presented with the polypoid adenoma data for formaldehyde might conclude that the experiment should be repeated. The policy maker may feel that he does not have time for that luxury.

Benzene. As we explained in Chapter 5, benzene has been shown to be a multipotential carcinogen in rats and mice. The key studies by Maltoni, the National Toxicology Program, and Goldstein provide twenty-three data sets—each representing a unique combination of species, sex, and tumor type. Which data set should be used to estimate human risk? Federal guidelines generally call for selection of the most sensitive species to predict human risk,[45] to allow for the possibility that humans are as sensitive as the most sensitive species tested.

Following the spirit of federal guidelines, the California DHS—which was estimating the human cancer risk of ambient benzene exposures in the ppb range—chose male mice as the relevant species and squamous cell carcinoma of the preputial gland as the relevant tumor type. This data set was selected because it was judged to be the most sensitive site in the more sensitive sex of the most sensitive species tested.

EPA guidelines seem to support this practice: "Because it is possible that human sensitivity is as high as the most sensitive responding animal species, in the absence of evidence to the contrary, the biologically acceptable data set from long-term studies showing the greatest sensitivity should generally be given the greatest emphasis, again with due regard to biological and statistical considerations."[46] The resulting human risk estimate, based on the linearized multistage model, was eight times higher than an estimate of leukemia risk at the same dose derived from the one-hit model and the Pliofilm workers' data.[47]

Critics argue that the sensitivity guideline is inappropriate in the case of benzene. Humans do not have a preputial gland, and even female mice did not show significant increases in such tumors after exposure to benzene. Thus, critics contend, use of the male mice data is likely to overstate human risk substantially.

The other major benzene risk assessment based on animal data was performed by Crump and Allen. Crump happens to be a key proponent of the multistage model and an advocate of uniform risk assessment guidelines.[48] Yet when faced with the benzene bioassay data, he and his colleague did not select the most sensitive response in animals. Instead they decided "to use data on leukemia whenever available, since this is the response noted in humans."[49] Maltoni's benzene-exposed rats, however, developed lymphoreticular leukemias, which are a subtype not associated with benzene in humans. Moreover, Crump and Allen used Goldstein's leukemia responses, even though the incidence of myelogenous leukemia he found was not statistically significantly increased relative to controls. The species they chose—rats and mice—in fact are known to be fairly insensitive to benzene-induced leukemia.

In an alternative analysis Crump and Allen examined all squamous cell carcinomas in male rats and male mice. The response in male mice is among the most sensitive, but it is not *the* most sensitive. They defended their choice by stating that "it is a more general response" than the preputial gland response and by noting that the upper confidence limits for the most sensitive responses were similar. The MLE, though, is about 2.3 times greater when the data on preputial gland tumors are selected instead of the data on combined squamous cell carcinomas.

This example raises a still more general issue. If several groups of animals, both males and females, of different species, are exposed to a chemical, several different carcinogenic responses may be analyzed in each group. As the number of dose-response relationships analyzed rises, it becomes increasingly likely that some groups, through chance, will exhibit an extremely high response rate. Thus, basing risk estimation on the "most sensitive" response involves a substantial probability of overestimating the risk because an effect that is inflated by a substantial random component is counted as "real."

Crump and Allen also differ from the California DHS in the factors used to convert mouse doses to human doses. The "scaling factor" employed by the California group, which is based upon body surface area, yields a twelve-fold greater risk than that calculated by Crump and Allen, who use a scaling factor based on relative body weight. No one knows which approach is more likely to be accurate.

The benzene analyses also reveal a counterintuitive point about the relationship between "information" and "uncertainty" in risk assessment. We often assume that more information reduces uncertainty. Yet here the availability of data from several animal bioassays appears to have increased the range of plausible risk estimates.

One reason that the animal tests on benzene have not done more to inform risk-assessment calculations is that the different bioassays have been performed for subtly, but importantly, different reasons. Goldstein's group is especially interested in developing a rodent model for chemical leukemogenesis. Maltoni is an experimentalist primarily interested in inducing tumors of any kind in test animals with chemicals that have tested negative in the hands of others. Even the NTP is not primarily concerned with translation to the human situation: their bioassay of benzene, like most chemicals they test, is by gavage (stomach tube), and this route of administration is usually discounted as a basis for inferring human risk from inhalation. If any of the three investigators had been primarily concerned with the regulatory policy questions, they might have examined inhalation at lower exposure levels and placed disproportionately more animals at these lower levels, but they did not.

This brief review also shows us that the question of what to do with positive animal data when imperfect yet positive human data are available cannot be resolved in a predetermined way by rigid general guidelines. It is all too possible that the case at hand will not fit the presumptions used when those guidelines were developed. Instead, conscientious risk assessment requires careful judgments about how best to characterize the total configuration of evidence. But the use of judgment raises still other problems, which we discuss in Chapter 7.

▪ Defining Dose

Dose is not a single number but rather multidimensional. Scientists simplify the notion to facilitate their inquiries, and risk assessors also do this regularly, but that does not mean such simplifications are persuasive. The difference between peak and intermittent exposures in carcinogenesis and the relationship between administered doses of a substance and the delivered or effective doses to target tissues both illustrate this problem.

Peak versus Cumulative Dose

The general practice of federal agencies is to assume that cumulative lifetime dose of a substance is the biologically relevant measure for human exposure.[50] But as we saw in Chapters 3 and 5, this practice may conceal much information and much uncertainty about carcinogenesis.

For example, some studies in animals indicate that high concentrations of formaldehyde over short periods of time are more toxic than lower concentrations over longer periods. Rats experienced much more irritation from exposures to 12 ppm formaldehyde for 3 hours than 3 ppm formaldehyde for 12 hours. The total dose was the same in the two cases—36 ppm hours—but it seems that cumulative dose was not the most relevant parameter. Irritation, though, may be more sensitive to concentration than is carcinogenesis. The laboratory animal bioassays for carcinogenesis were performed according to standard protocols and hence involved continuous exposure for six hours per day, five days per week. It is not known what effect administering the same total ppm hours of formaldehyde over either shorter or longer intervals would have had on the tumor rates. For other chemicals the evidence is mixed. For vinyl chloride, peak exposures of short duration appear to be most carcinogenic to humans. Yet in laboratory animals long-term exposures to low levels of vinyl chloride are much more tumorigenic than brief exposures to peak levels.[51] For formaldehyde, though, a plausible argument can be made that carcinogenic response will be more dependent upon concentration than upon cumulative amount.

This issue has obvious policy relevance because humans exposed to formaldehyde in the workplace are more likely to be exposed on an intermittent basis. This is certainly the case for morticians, who probably spend one or two hours a day actually embalming and the other hours of the workday with little or no exposure to formaldehyde.

Risk assessors have nonetheless tended to compute average aggregate exposures to formaldehyde. For example, EPA analysts divide formaldehyde exposure by time to calculate an "averaged daily exposure."[52] Although this method is mathematically convenient, some scientists consider these conversions to be contrary to evidence and intuition. The method implies that the pathologist exposed to 1 ppm of formaldehyde for 1 hour every day is at the same risk as the individual who spends 24 hours inside a UFFI home with an ambient formaldehyde level of 0.05 ppm. Many scientists would not equate these two situations because they believe that higher concentrations produce disproportionately greater effects.

Deciding what parameters of dose are relevant to response has implications for regulatory policy that are much broader than issues of the reliability of quantitative risk estimates. In particular, should the policy debate be about whether the occupational standard for the TWA is too high, or should it also be about whether the ceilings, or peak exposures, should come down? Some analysts maintain that the worker most likely to be at risk of adverse health effects is the one who sustains a half-hour exposure to 5 or more ppm—even if he received virtually no additional exposure to formaldehyde. His co-worker exposed to 0.5 ppm for ten times as long may be at a much lower risk. Yet these complexities have been generally omitted from the quantitative risk assessments.

As we noted in Chapter 3, not all mechanistic arguments lead to lower risk estimates. Nor do alternatives to cumulative dose as an exposure measure always lead to lower human risk estimates. In particular, Hattis and coworkers predicted human risks from formaldehyde on the basis of dose *rate* rather than an integrated amount. Although the results are similar to those of other models at the upper confidence limits, the midrange estimates are substantially larger for most exposure patterns. Their midrange projection of excess cancers among U.S. workers for prevailing formaldehyde exposures is about 1,000 *per year*. In contrast, the number of excess occupational cancers from the multistage model is, according to one study, about 70 cases for exposed workers observed for a *lifetime*.[53]

Although the model used by Hattis and coworkers has been criticized as being too theoretical and having a relatively poor fit with the CIIT data, the point is that it is not certain that any given approach will always be the most conservative possible. Another model can almost always be postulated that will produce still larger estimated cancer risks.

In their risk assessment of benzene, Crump and Allen also probed the adequacy of various measures of dose from the epidemiology studies. They looked at such measures as cumulative exposure, weighted cumulative exposure, "windows" of exposure, and peak exposures. Their work revealed that peak exposures were no more predictive of risk than were cumulative exposures: "This analysis does not support the hypothesis that peak exposure [benzene concentrations greater than 76 ppm] has any effect upon risk over that which can be explained by the contribution of these exposures to cumulative dose. If anything, it suggests that high exposures are less effective per ppm-year in producing leukemia than lower exposures."[54] This would seem to refute some views of biological mechanisms that were discussed in Chapter 5. Since the subset of workers exposed to high peaks significantly overlaps that subset exposed to large cumulative amounts, the data are limited in their ability to address the hypothesis.

Administered versus Delivered Doses

A second problem with standard risk estimates is that they assume that the administered dose of a chemical in a laboratory animal bioassay is proportional to the delivered dose to target tissues. This assumption may oftentimes be wrong. As we noted in Chapter 3, some experimental evidence shows that the rate of covalent binding of formaldehyde to respiratory epithelial DNA is about four times lower at 2 ppm than what would be predicted from the finding at higher levels of exposure. Table 6.6 shows how the use of these data can change estimated risks at low doses. The MLEs of cancer risk based upon delivered dose for low levels of formaldehyde exposure are about two orders of magnitude smaller than the risks predicted from corresponding administered doses, assuming the multistage model is used.[55] And plausible biological mechanisms have been offered to explain this result.[56]

These risk estimates, if biologically accurate, have profound policy implications. They suggest that the low doses of formaldehyde that are of concern to CPSC or EPA do not pose a significant risk to humans. As we noted in Chapter 3, the use of such delivered-dose data in quantitative risk assessment raises important issues of

Table 6.6 Formaldehyde risk estimates: administered (A) versus delivered (D) doses.[a]

		Excess lifetime cancer risk	
Concentration (ppm)	*Dose measure*	*MLE*	*UCL*
1.0	A	2.5×10^{-4}	1.8×10^{-3}
	D	4.7×10^{-6}	6.24×10^{-4}
0.5	A	3.4×10^{-5}	8.09×10^{-4}
	D	5.8×10^{-7}	3.10×10^{-4}
0.1	A	2.51×10^{-7}	1.56×10^{-4}
	D	4.70×10^{-9}	6.19×10^{-5}

Source: T. B. Starr and R. D. Buck, "The Importance of Delivered Dose in Estimating Low-Dose Cancer Risk from Inhalation Exposure to Formaldehyde," *Fundamentals of Applied Toxicology,* 4 (1984): 740–753.

a. Estimates are based on the multistage model with a third-degree polynomial.

precedent—which in turn generates strategic behavior by pro- and anti-regulation forces.

Skeptics of this approach emphasize that such "pharmacokinetic" models "tend to be considerably less conservative than the currently accepted low-dose extrapolation models without having been demonstrated to be biologically accurate."[57] In particular, DNA-adduct formation has not been shown to be the "sole mechanism" of formaldehyde's carcinogenicity. And there is no data on the ratio of administered to delivered dose of formaldehyde in humans—which is hardly surprising since scientists do not even know what the target tissues and organs in humans are.

• Conclusion

The approach to quantification of cancer risk promoted by EPA's Carcinogen Assessment Group (GLOBAL 79 and GLOBAL 82) is now available in computer software and has become widely used. The method is based on the following combination of conservative assessment guidelines: no thresholds in dose-response functions; linearity in the dose-response function at low doses; cumulative lifetime exposure as the measure of dose; a presumed proportional relationship between administered and delivered doses, even at low levels; inclusion of benign tumors in dose-response estimation, unless there is compelling information to the contrary, and use of the most sensitive animal species as the basis for extrapolation of cancer risk to humans. Very little technical discretion has been delegated to the scientists interested in toxicology; generic guidelines have been devised to resolve most questions of judgment, interpretation, and extrapolation.

Because cancer risk estimates appear to play a critical role in setting priorities and standards, it is not surprising that federal agencies have sought to dictate the proper practice of risk assessment. Permitting members of the scientific community outside of federal agencies to make case-by-case risk estimates for various chemicals would be— given the large uncertainties about low-dose risks—tantamount to relinquishing control over the regulatory process. Standardized methodology was clearly planned to keep control of priority setting and standard setting in the hands of regulators.

The widespread and increasing reliance on CAG's risk-assessment methodology might not be troubling if we could be sure that agency risk assessors would receive timely feedback from scientists about the adequacy of their algorithms, and that they would adjust their assumptions over time to reflect reality. Even if we knew that current estimates of cancer risk were in error, we might be reassured if we knew that these forecasts would be revised as necessary in the future.

But here is a key problem. It is very unlikely that agency risk assessors will receive any timely feedback from scientific research about the properties (for example, accuracy and variance) of their low-dose risk estimates. Laboratory animal bioassays and epidemiological studies generally lack the statistical power to support or refute the predictions of low-dose cancer risk that are of concern to policy makers. In the case of formaldehyde, even a relatively large-scale epidemiological investigation such as the one completed by the National Cancer Institute, was too insensitive to either detect or refute some of the human risk estimates that agencies projected from the CIIT bioassay data. For benzene, the rarity of leukemia means that scientists may never be able to discern whether lowering OSHA's PEL from 10 to 1 ppm actually causes a decline in the incidence of leukemia among exposed workers. Unlike the performance of weathermen or econometric forecasters, the performance of cancer risk assessors cannot usually be objectively evaluated.

Our view is that risk assessment has become too formalized and mechanical in light of the limited data. Little is gained from the sophisticated massaging of weak data. The key challenge is to improve the quality of the data used in risk assessment. But how can this be done if direct measurement of the relevant risks is impractical or impossible? As we shall argue in Chapter 7, the answer lies partly in developing a better understanding of the mechanisms that produce cancer and partly in eliciting careful scientific judgments. Better information on mechanisms might allow extrapolation to be performed more intelligently on a chemical-by-chemical basis. Giving the judgments of working scientists a greater role in risk assessment would allow for revision of estimates that go against scientific intuition.

Society must face a large and irreducible element of uncertainty in the estimation of cancer risk. No amount of data on the mechanisms of carcinogenesis or scientific intuition can substitute for direct observation of low-dose effects in humans. The uncertainties—both those that are reducible and those that are inevitable—need to be acknowledged and (when possible) quantified by risk assessors. Otherwise, policy makers and the public will be misled.

7 ▪ SCIENCE AND POLICY CONFLICT

MANY PEOPLE look to further scientific research to fill the gaps in our understanding of carcinogenicity and thus resolve policy conflicts. In this chapter we offer some general observations and recommendations about the role of science in the regulatory process. We refer back to the case studies of formaldehyde and benzene, not because they are representative of all regulatory experience, but because, as we noted in Chapter 1, they illustrate the central problems confronting regulatory agencies and the scientific community. Our case studies suggest, somewhat surprisingly, that at least so far scientific research has exacerbated policy disagreements as often as it has resolved them. And this situation is not likely to change soon.

▪ The Limits of Science

Regulators are asking increasingly sophisticated and quantitative questions of scientists. OSHA asks whether exposing a worker to formaldehyde concentrations of 1 ppm for thirty-five years will increase his or her chances of contracting cancer by more than 1 in 1,000. EPA wants to know how many additional cases of cancer will occur among a population of one million residents who are exposed to 10 ppb of benzene for a seventy-year lifetime. CPSC seeks to determine how much a person's probability of contracting cancer is elevated by living for ten years in a house insulated with urea-formaldehyde foam.

One of the most important, albeit discouraging, findings of the case studies is that the available scientific data seldom allow scientists to confidently answer such questions. The principal methods of inquiry—epidemiology, laboratory animal bioassays, and mutagenicity tests—simply do not provide reliable estimates of the increase in human cancer that will result from chronic low-level chemical exposures. A brief review of the strengths and limitations of these methods shows this very clearly.

Epidemiology

The basic strategy of cancer epidemiology is to compare cancer mortality among individuals exposed to a chemical to those rates among an apparently similar group of individuals who have not been exposed. This traditional cohort design has successfully detected the carcinogenic effects of tobacco smoke, asbestos, vinyl chloride, and roughly twenty other chemicals and mixtures.[1] Positive findings from a cohort study are especially persuasive when it can be shown that cancer rates increase as exposure levels rise. This makes it less likely (although not impossible) that differences between the exposed and unexposed groups are the result of chance or some confounding factor.

In the case of benzene, for example, the epidemiology provided convincing qualitative evidence that high levels of benzene exposure among workers caused an increase in the incidence of leukemia. Describing the dose-response relationship quantitatively, however, has proven to be extremely difficult. The clinical studies by Aksoy and Vigliani could not satisfy this need because they did not have reliable exposure data and they did not have a control group or other evidence of the background rate of leukemia among comparable unexposed individuals. Indeed, they did not really have a cohort at all since they neither studied nor knew the size of the entire exposed population. As a result, they did not even know the rate of disease in that population.

The studies of benzene by Infante, Ott, and Shell were much more complete, but they too lacked reliable exposure data. Furthermore, what imprecise evidence there was on exposures suggests that the concentrations were quite high relative to the levels that regulatory agencies are currently interested in. None of the studies provide direct evidence about the effects of chronic benzene exposures in the range of 1 ppb to 10 ppm—the concern in contemporary policy debates. As long as scientists have no reliable way to fill in the gaps left by the missing data, any estimates are necessarily arbitrary and entail controversial and uncertain extrapolation.

The epidemiological studies of formaldehyde encountered additional, but not unusual, problems. The incidence of nasal cancer (the response observed in rodents) is so rare in humans that it cannot be profitably studied within a cohort design. The study population would have to be too large. Instead Olsen attempted a case-control study, in which a group of patients with a specific disease is compared with a group suffering from some other disease. This approach gives enough cases but raises the problem of whether the controls differ only in the exposure being studied. Olsen encountered this problem when he discovered that the workers exposed to formaldehyde had also been exposed to wood dust, a known nasal tumorigen. The cohort studies of formaldehyde and lung cancer were also plagued by a serious and uncontrolled confounder: cigarette smoking. The epidemiological studies of formaldehyde also suffered to a greater or lesser extent from the same problem of poor information about exposures that plagued the benzene epidemiology.

Perhaps the most serious limitation of all the epidemiology we reviewed was its limited statistical power and hence its limited capacity to detect relatively low risks of cancer. Even if historical exposure data are accurate and confounders nonexistent, epidemiological methods generally cannot detect 1 in 1,000 to 1 in 1,000,000 lifetime risks. Our calculations in Chapter 3 revealed that even the NCI's relatively large study of formaldehyde-exposed workers was incapable of detecting the policy-relevant risk levels predicted from extrapolations from the CIIT's rat study.

The limited capacity of epidemiology to detect effects means that negative results are not unlikely, even when the chemical is a genuine human carcinogen. This possibility further confuses the interpretation of any studies that are available. Are negative results "real" in this case, or are they the result of low statistical power? Although negative epidemiological findings can sometimes place a useful upper bound on excess human cancer risk, these upper bounds will generally be above the minimum risk levels of concern to regulators.

Laboratory Animal Bioassays

When nature and history design "poor" experiments, scientists commonly resort to laboratory animal bioassays. Rodents are usually used because they are small, reproduce rapidly, and have relatively short lifetimes. They are less expensive to purchase and maintain—using less space, time, and food—than larger animals. Several hundred chemicals and mixtures have already been shown by toxicologists to cause cancer in animals.[2] All of the twenty or so known human carcinogens except arsenic have also been shown to cause cancer in at least one site in animals.

Nonetheless, inferring human cancer risk from carcinogenic responses in animals has some inherent uncertainties. Rodents and humans differ in physiology and metabolic processes. Also, for practical reasons, scientists often expose rodents to much larger doses than those of interest to regulators. Finally, practical constraints on experimentation cause the conditions of exposure in laboratory settings to be imperfect simulations of real-world human exposures.

Our case studies reveal all three problems. First, and most obvious, is the problem of interspecies extrapolation. Rodents and humans are not always equally sensitive to the carcinogenic effects of a chemical. Although almost all known human carcinogens are animal carcinogens, the target organs frequently vary across species, and scientists do not yet know what proportion of animal carcinogens are human carcinogens. Benzene is known to be a leukemogen in humans but apparently is not in rodents. There are also differences between animal species. When the same concentrations of formaldehyde were administered to rats and mice, the rats responded with a much higher incidence of nasal tumors than the mice. Which animal model is the "correct" basis for forecasting human responses? Since toxicologists cannot generally verify their animal findings in humans, they cannot confidently answer regulators' questions.

Second, the high-to-low-dose extrapolation problem encountered with epidemiological data occurs here as well. In order to produce enough tumors to analyze, experimenters have to either greatly increase the number of treated animals or raise the dose to which each animal is exposed. The former strategy may be too expensive, while the latter strategy, which is common practice, leaves unanswered the question of how the responses observed at high doses should be extrapolated to low doses.

Finally, the route of administration used by experimenters is not necessarily identical to the route of exposure of concern to regulators. Although it is easier for experimenters to precisely control dosage when rodents are exposed to chemicals by stomach tube, it may be difficult to relate the responses to potential human risk from inhalation or ingestion. The responses observed in Maltoni's initial animal bioassay of benzene were difficult to interpret because the chemical was administered by gavage, though his findings were later confirmed by inhalation experiments. A more subtle route-of-administration problem surfaced with formaldehyde because rats, unlike humans, are obligate nose breathers.

Mutagenicity Tests

Because of the time and expense associated with long-term animal tests, regulators have paid increasing attention to short-term tests on cultured cells to provide some "quick and dirty" assessments. Short-term tests for mutagenesis provide information on the potential of a chemical to interact with DNA. Experimental evidence also indicates that chemicals that can damage DNA are likely to be carcinogens, though the correlation is far from perfect. Benzene, for example, is a known carcinogen yet is not a mutagen. Moreover, interpreting these tests is made more difficult by the possibility that some carcinogens are epigenetic and thus do not act through pathways that involve genetic alterations, a hypothesis that has been advanced for both benzene and formaldehyde.

Our case studies suggest that the results of mutagenicity tests are not very important to the regulatory process when positive epidemiology or positive animal tests are available. The epidemiological findings linking benzene to leukemia were sufficient to create regulatory concern, even though mutagenicity tests were negative. Likewise, the results of CIIT's formaldehyde bioassay were sufficient to trigger regulatory controversy, even though mutagenicity tests of formaldehyde had produced mixed results. Even if benzene and formaldehyde had been shown to be potent mutagens, it is not clear that this fact alone—without positive data from animal or human tests—would have been sufficient to create policy pressures.

Mutagenicity information does play a role in scientific discussions about the low-dose risks of carcinogens. Some scientists regard positive mutagenicity tests as an indication that a carcinogen is likely to be genotoxic and hence to be characterized by a linear dose-response curve at low levels. Benzene is not considered to be a classical carcinogen by some in part because of the negative mutagenicity information. Other scientists are skeptical about whether any reliable information about low-dose cancer risks can be inferred from short-term tests. They are particularly unconvinced that chemicals can be classified as "strong" or "weak" mutagens on the basis of such tests in a way that is relevant to forecasting human risk. In any case, the current state of the art in short-term tests does not provide the regulator with what he or she ultimately wants: quantification of the low-dose risks of chemical carcinogens.

▪ Sources of Scientific Conflict

Since neither epidemiology nor nonhuman studies yield direct evidence on the low-dose carcinogenic effects of chemicals, those who would estimate such effects must fall back on theories and models. Hence we have observed a burgeoning interest in quantitative risk assessment and a large and controversial literature about how to do it.[3] As scientists move from data to extrapolation, from evidence to speculation, the opportunities for scientific conflicts multiply.

These conflicts are exacerbated by the pressure from regulatory institutions. Without such pressure, the limits on scientific knowledge would not be of much significance, for scientists would patiently wait for better data. However, because cancer is a dread disease and because some chemicals have been implicated as causative agents, citizens have used the legislative and political process to insist that steps be taken to protect public health. As a result, regulatory choices have to be made today on the available, less-than-perfect information. As this process unfolds, scientists are asked to offer their advice despite the substantial technical uncertainties.

As scientists have participated in the rulemaking process, disagreements, often heated, have occurred. To the ordinary citizen these disagreements are bound to be somewhat bewildering. Although it is no surprise that groups with particular economic or ideological interests seek to recruit scientists to their side of the policy debate, it is not obvious why scientists should disagree as much as they appear to about what are presumably matters of science.

Confusing Questions Posed by Regulators

Early concern about chemicals and cancer led to questions such as, "Is this chemical a carcinogen?" That is the question asked by the Delaney Amendment to the Food, Drug, and Cosmetic Act of 1958.[4] The question is also quite central to implementation of the generic cancer policies developed in the 1970s by OSHA, EPA, and CPSC.

But scientists have trouble answering such a question because the terminology is too simplistic. Should formaldehyde be considered a carcinogen in humans based on the experimental findings in rodents, even though the epidemiological findings are at best ambiguous? Should benzene be considered a carcinogen at low exposure levels even though some scientists suspect that the positive epidemiological findings at high levels are attributable to acute bone marrow toxicity that does not occur at low doses? The answers to these questions are in dispute, in part because the questions are not precise from a scientist's point of view, so the scientists who try to answer them must formulate their own definitions of a carcinogen for policy purposes.

A slightly different question is "What is a safe dose for a suspected chemical carcinogen?" This is the question implicit in all laws and rules that require public officials to set a standard that provides "safety." We found a more elaborate version of this approach in section 112 of the Clean Air Act Amendments of 1970, which directs EPA to set emission standards for "hazardous air pollutants" that protect the public health with "an ample margin of safety."[5]

These policy formulations are bound to generate scientific conflict because certain theories of chemical carcinogenesis imply there is no safe level; instead they presume that some risk is associated with any dose of a carcinogen.[6] Indeed, this is the unproven yet unrefuted assumption behind the one-hit and linearized multistage models of risk assessment commonly used by federal agencies. As long as the questions posed by regulators start with a premise that not all scientists share (that "safety" or an "ample margin of safety" is possible), we can expect scientists to offer conflicting responses.

In the Supreme Court's handling of the 1980 benzene case, Justice Stevens offered another formulation of the regulatory question. OSHA, said Justice Stevens, must determine that a chemical poses a significant risk of cancer before initiating a rulemaking. Focusing regulatory attention on the magnitude of risk instead of its mere existence is a more sophisticated approach. Still more sophisticated is the doctrine of unreasonable risk that supposedly governs the rulemaking activities of CPSC and EPA under the Toxic Substances Control Act. This doctrine calls for balancing the magnitude of cancer risk—assuming it can somehow be quantified by scientists—against the dangers and costs of regulation.

There is a paradox in the growing subtlety of regulators' questions about chemical carcinogens. On the one hand, when very simple questions are asked, the conscientious scientist finds it difficult to know how to answer because of the ambiguity created by simplification. On the other hand, scientific knowledge is not adequate to answer the more elaborate questions with any measure of confidence. Our point is that scientists often seem to disagree with one another because they are caught between ambiguity and ignorance, between questions that are too hard and questions that are too simple.

Different Implicit Burdens of Proof

These conflicts over how scientists should respond to regulators when knowledge is limited become particularly acute when there are also disagreements over where to place the burden of proof in various arguments. Our case studies reveal that conflicts among scientists often arise—sometimes unknowingly—from different answers to these kinds of questions.

The varied interpretations of the original CIIT formaldehyde bioassay are a case in point. The nonlinearity in the observed dose-response points was interpreted by some analysts as a hint that low levels of exposure to formaldehyde are associated with little or no excess cancer risk. Others argued that the threshold hypothesis was not proven and that regulators should not assume the existence of a no-effect exposure level until compelling evidence suggests otherwise.

When CIIT later published information on the amount of inhaled formaldehyde that is delivered to DNA in the rat's nasal lining, a similar dispute emerged. Contrary to the proportional relationship typically assumed in risk assessment, CIIT investigators found that the dose delivered to DNA diminished rapidly as the amount of formaldehyde inhaled by rats declined. A panel of scientists appointed by EPA concluded that it was premature for EPA to utilize the delivered-dose information in risk assessment because of various experimental problems of internal and external validity. CIIT scientists argued in contrast that their experiments were persuasive enough to shift the burden of proof to those who wanted a constant proportionality between administered and delivered dose.

We believe that this dispute is a harbinger of things to come. As more mechanistic data of this sort become available, they are likely to generate more disputes. Questions will be raised about whether the information is precise or reliable enough to replace the traditonal—and presumably more conservative—assumptions that normally govern risk assessment.

Similar difficulties arise concerning what statistical test to use when analyzing experimental results. Classical statistical methods are designed to minimize the likelihood of "type I error" (accepting new hypotheses that are in fact false) even at the cost of a high probability of "type II error" (rejecting a true new idea for lack of sufficient evidence).[7] But just how much proof should be required before a result is called statistically significant? Indeed, how do we decide which of several alternative ideas is to get the benefit of the doubt—is to be given the status of the null hypothesis that is presumed to be true until disproven? Differences of opinion on these points are also a fertile source of scientific conflict.

This problem is illustrated in our case studies by the varying interpretations that scientists gave to the statistically insignificant number of mouse nasal tumors in the formaldehyde experiments. Calling them "biologically significant" was a way for some scientists to say that the numbers were informative, despite the lack of statistical significance at the arbitrary level of confidence initially specified by the investigators. A minority argued that their statistical insignificance was the important point.

• Differences in Scientific Interpretation

Scientists' disciplinary backgrounds and general theoretical views also influence their approaches to questions and to evidence. This can lead both to divergent interpretations of specific data and to different approaches to combining diverse sources of information. As a result, even within their domain of expertise, scientists disagree about answers to the questions posed by regulators.

Consider, for example, how often the epidemiological findings that we have reviewed have been subject to divergent interpretations. Some scientists interpreted Acheson's study of formaldehyde as negative, while others drew attention to the excess number of lung cancers among blue-collar workers exposed to formaldehyde at a particular plant. Wong's study of benzene-exposed workers was interpreted in one way by those who compared the observed leukemia rate to the low rate in the control group of workers and in another way by those who contrasted that same rate with the higher overall rate in the general population.

Animal studies also provide ample room for variation in scientific judgment. Pathologists had some difficulty distinguishing benign tumors (polypoid adenomas) from metaplasia in the CIIT formaldehyde bioassay, and various analysts took the presence of benign tumors more or less seriously. Some took seriously, and others not, the lack of a dose-response relationship for the benign tumors, while others emphasized the difference in cell type between the benign and the malignant tumors. Or consider how the toxicological meaning of malignant tumors in the Zymbal gland of rodents—a gland with no obvious human counterpart—was disputed after publication of Maltoni's bioassay of benzene.

Such conflict is especially likely to occur when diverse sources of information lead to different implications for potential human risk. Having given more weight to CIIT's animal data than to the inconclusive human data, Upton and others saw formaldehyde as a potentially serious carcinogenic threat to humans. Higginson and coworkers, in contrast, were less impressed with the rat data and took some comfort in the apparently negative epidemiology.

Similarly, because benzene is considered a proven human and animal carcinogen, many scientists believe that any dose presents a carcinogenic risk to humans. Others are less certain because there is no good animal model of benzene's leukemogenic effects. They see the negative mutagenicity tests and the toxic effects of benzene on the bone marrow as indications that the chemical is not a classical carcinogen. As a consequence, they take seriously the possibility that it operates through an epigenetic process and that there might be a threshold in the dose-response function.

Such differences are often exacerbated by differences in disciplinary training. In the example just mentioned, the clinical hematologists seemed to find the notion of a threshold response more plausible than did the quantitative risk assessors, whose methods generally presume nonthreshold responses. Someone whose entire training has been oriented toward finding a safe level is likely to see that idea supported by the data. A discipline-based dispute was also apparent in the formaldehyde controversy, where the epidemiologists seemed less persuaded of the potential for human risk than the toxicologists, in part because the data produced by the toxicologists' methods pointed that way, while the studies by epidemiologists were generally inconclusive.

Scientists also may hold very different general theoretical beliefs—in our case, conflicting ideas about the process of carcinogenesis. Those who take seriously epigenetic theories of carcinogenesis were inclined to interpret the formaldehyde and benzene data as consistent with these theories. They saw formaldehyde acting as a carcinogen only through the irritation resulting from relatively high exposure levels. The nonlinear dose-response points in the CIIT rat bioassay were viewed as consistent with an epigenetic mechanism. This group recognized benzene as a leukemogen but believed that in this case the disease was only an outgrowth of bone marrow toxicity from high exposure levels.

In contrast, scientists who emphasize genotoxic theories of carcinogenesis did not see formaldehyde or benzene as exceptions. For them, formaldehyde's mutagenic potential meant that it might well cause cancer through DNA-related pathways at low exposure levels. Similarly, once benzene was shown to produce solid tumors at multiple sites in multiple species, those who viewed carcinogens as generally genotoxic were reinforced in their view that benzene too operated in this way.

In all of these examples, correct answers were elusive. The frontiers of science are often ambiguous, and disagreements are not readily resolved by objective or even consensual means. Instead, intuition, craftsmanship, and judgment are critical. Thus whenever we ask science at the frontier to play a role in regulatory policy, we must expect the kinds of disagreements we have seen.

Influence of Policy Beliefs

When public policy is an issue, additional problems arise in interpreting and using scientific knowledge. Scientists, like other citizens, may hold strong policy views that can influence their evaluations of particular studies.

Admittedly it is often impossible to know for certain when policy concerns are influencing scientific judgment. We nonetheless did see some apparent instances of such strategic behavior. In particular, the debates between Infante's group and Lamm and Wilson about the Pliofilm study and benzene's leukemogenic effects seem to have been exacerbated and polarized by the regulatory context. In a different way, the heated dispute between Cohn and coworkers and the Casanova-Schmitz group about formaldehyde was apparently influenced by policy pressures. Both sides viewed the acceptability of the delivered-dose data on formaldehyde as a precedent-setting issue, with policy implications well beyond the formaldehyde rulemakings. When scientific findings are closely linked to policy action, the differences in scientists' interpretations are likely to be polarized and hardened.

▪ Scientific Research, Knowledge, and Policy Conflict

Our examination of the disputes about formaldehyde and benzene shows that the "static hypothesis"—that scientists can settle their disagreements about the available data and thereby settle policy disputes about human risk at low doses—is not necessarily confirmed by experience. Still, many people continue to hope that current disagreements can and will be narrowed by additional research. This might be called the "dynamic hypothesis." The hope is that larger studies, or different types of studies, or better modeling based on existing data will generate knowledge that can help resolve both scientific and policy conflicts. In Figure 7.1, which depicts research, knowledge, and policy conflict as a three-dimensional space, this notion is represented by the arrow labeled (A). (The term "knowledge" is problematical, as we shall explain shortly.) The claim is that more research, which policy makers could stimulate, will lead to more knowledge and in turn to less policy conflict. In fact our cases provide a good deal of evidence about this dynamic hypothesis, and much of it contradicts this apparently plausible assertion.

One way to explore this notion is to assign particular scientific studies of formaldehyde and benzene to cells in a two-by-three matrix (see Figure 7.2). Assigning a study to a cell requires judgments about whether the study generated significant knowledge and whether it influenced policy conflict. According to the dynamic hypothesis, we should find most studies in the right-hand box in the bottom row (more knowledge, less conflict), with perhaps a few unsuccessful studies in the left and center boxes in the top row. We were intrigued to discover that, as we will show, we could find examples of studies

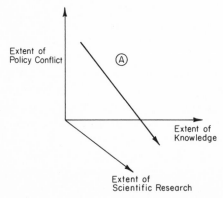

7.1   The effects of scientific research on knowledge and policy conflict.

	More Policy Conflict	No Effect on Policy Conflict	Less Policy Conflict
No More Knowledge			
More Knowledge			

7.2 Potential effects of scientific research on knowledge and policy conflict.

in all of these boxes. There was no consistent positive relationship between either research and knowledge or knowledge and policy agreement.

Before going further, we consider what we mean by knowledge, belief, and consensus, and how these concepts interrelate. We are acutely conscious of the arguments of Thomas Kuhn and his successors and critics to the effect that scientific "knowledge" is definable only in relation to a larger conceptual framework of both substantive and methodological theories. Furthermore, we realize that to say knowledge is advanced when theories "fit" the facts "better" begs certain key questions. Scientists must decide what criteria to use to measure fit. And there is always the possibility that the relative rankings of various competing scientific ideas may, at any one time, vary with the criteria chosen. Indeed, another way to talk about some of the disputes we have reviewed—such as those over risk assessment methods—is to see these as disputes over criteria.

Nevertheless, our epistemological position is at root what philosophers call realism. We do believe there is an external world and that human knowledge of it can be improved, even though we must do so through the mediating process of concepts and theories and by using evaluatory criteria that are our own creation. Furthermore, in the world of contemporary biomedical science, there is enough epistemological agreement at the most fundamental level that accumulating evidence of an accepted sort typically will convince most scientists that one view is superior in relation to another view. Thus when we use the term "knowledge" we mean "that which most of the relevant scientists have come to accept as a better account of the world in the medium run." By "medium run" we mean longer than one month and less than ten years, to allow for communication, cogitation, and confirmation; we recognize that in the long run ideas are likely to be superseded by still other, different "knowledge." Thus we are compelled to use the "medium-run" widespread acceptance of an idea by the scientific community as a test of whether it is in fact a contribution to knowledge.

In taking this position, however, we are hardly asserting that what constitutes "real" knowledge either can be or is likely to be agreed to by all participants in a particular policy dispute—especially in the heat of battle. On the contrary, we have repeatedly stressed that a number of factors, from training and professional ambition to consciousness of social consequences, may influence how scientists react to new studies. And much of the resulting disagreement will be framed in terms of the believability (or even the "truth") of various knowledge claims.

Hence some of the analysis we propose can only be done retrospectively, when "things have shaken down a bit." Furthermore, any one characterization of what occurred may never be acceptable to all of those who participated. We say this because we do not believe that we, or any other observer, can stand in some neutral or universal position outside the fray. Nevertheless, we believe that the idea of the knowledge conveyed by a study captures something very important about that study. And that something is also an unavoidable feature of any relevant account of the role of science in social conflict.

More Knowledge, More Policy Conflict

One of the central lessons of the formaldehyde case study is that additional knowledge can increase policy conflict. The obvious example is the CIIT bioassay, which was the first definitive demonstration that exposure to formaldehyde causes cancer in rodents.

Prior to the CIIT bioassay there was relatively little concern about the need to regulate human exposure to formaldehyde. Officials at CPSC and OSHA were somewhat concerned about the chemical's irritant effects, but no major regulatory decisions were imminent. It was the CIIT results—and the resulting possibility of human cancer risk—that stimulated serious regulatory pressures and deliberations. (This effect was magnified because the results were released at the same time that federal agencies were adopting generic guidelines to the effect that positive animal tests should be considered presumptive evidence of human cancer risk.)

Although CIIT's bioassay results were powerful enough to generate regulatory consideration of formaldehyde, there was no policy agreement about what to do about the human exposures under the jurisdiction of CPSC and EPA. CPSC's attempted ban of formaldehyde insulation was hotly contested by the Formaldehyde Institute and proved to be so highly controversial that it was ultimately overturned by a federal appeals court. EPA did not take any significant regulatory action on formaldehyde, despite seven years (1980–1986) of heated controversy and litigation. A major uncertainty facing regulators at both EPA and CPSC was the large discrepancy between the high concentrations of formaldehyde administered to rodents by CIIT scientists and the low levels of formaldehyde present in homes and ambient air. Thus a study that raised questions it could not answer (issues of low-dose human risk) served to increase policy conflict.

More Knowledge, Less Policy Conflict

To say that not all cases confirm the dynamic hypothesis does not mean that none do. On the contrary, the case studies provide several illustrations of scientific research creating knowledge that reduced policy conflict.

The formaldehyde bioassays by scientists at CIIT and NYU, combined with continuing concerns about irritation, were sufficient to persuade most of those involved in regulation that the OSHA standard for workplace exposure should be lowered. Unlike the situations at CPSC and EPA, the 3 ppm OSHA limit was very close to the exposure levels in the CIIT bioassay associated with excess tumors (2, 6, and 15 ppm). For tactical reasons the formaldehyde industry sought to persuade OSHA to tighten the standard based on irritation rather than on cancer risk. But even the key industry group, the Formaldehyde Institute, was ultimately supportive of a tighter occupational exposure standard. This example reveals another interesting point. The same study can lead to seemingly contradictory effects at different regulatory agencies, depending on the particular points at issue.

A second example of science producing consensual policy change was the work on benzene by Aksoy in Turkey and Vigliani in Italy. Their clinical observations of benzene-induced leukemia and aplastic anemia led to fairly rapid and major reductions in human exposures to benzene in their countries. Interestingly, their work was not as influential at U.S. companies and regulatory institutions.

Sometimes additional research changes the distribution of technical opinion without fully resolving the technical disagreements. Still, those changes in scientific beliefs can in turn have an effect on regulatory policy. Such seems to have been the case with the animal bioassays of benzene completed by Maltoni and the National Toxicology Program in the early 1980s. These results apparently played a role in increasing support for a reduction in OSHA's permissible exposure limit. The studies revealed excess cancers other than leukemia in exposed rats and mice. Since some reputable scientists were inclined to regard benzene-induced leukemia as an exclusively high-dose phenomenon related to bone marrow toxicity, the case for regulating low levels of benzene exposure had not been clear cut. Although some significant dissenters remained, the incidence of solid tumors that Maltoni observed lent credence to the view that benzene could be a classical carcinogen.

More Knowledge, No Effect on Policy Conflict

There are also examples of scientific research producing knowledge that has no effect on policy conflict, even though, on the face of it, the research seems quite relevant. Consider, for example, the experimental work on the toxicological effects of intermittent and peak exposures to benzene and formaldehyde. The implication of this research is that the time pattern of exposure is a biologically important parameter for determining cancer risks. Yet agency risk assessors and managers have traditionally assumed that the goal of standard setting is to reduce cumulative lifetime exposures, and most standard setting and risk assessment is done on that basis.

Although one might have expected this line of research to redefine policy conflict, it did not do so. The policy discussions about benzene at OSHA continued to be dominated by disagreement about how low to set the eight-hour TWA exposure limit. Less attention was given to limiting short-term exposures to control workers' peak exposures. Indeed, OSHA's original proposal to tighten the formaldehyde exposure rule contained a provision that would have deleted the existing short-term exposure limits. This incident reveals something important about the impact (or nonimpact) of science on policy disputes. When the bureaucratic and conceptual apparatus is oriented one way, technical work that suggests a recasting of the entire discussion may have a hard time being heard, especially when no advocacy group is supporting such a change in the deliberations.

No More Knowledge, More Policy Conflict

In all of the cases discussed thus far, it appears that additional research did produce additional knowledge. What about studies that do not add to knowledge? We have seen a variety of outcomes, including the distressing situation in which a study instigates a heated policy dispute without offering much in the way of knowledge. This can happen when an ambiguous result is seized on by one side to support a hypothesis with powerful regulatory implications, while others deny the relevance of the work.

Consider for example Infante and coworkers' study of excess leukemia among workers exposed to benzene in manufacturing Pliofilm. Viewed merely as confirmation of Aksoy and Vigliani's earlier clinical discoveries of benzene-induced leukemia, it would not have instigated much policy conflict. The controversy occurred when some tried to use the study as a basis for quantifying the dose-response relationship at the levels of exposure experienced by U.S. workers in the 1970s and 1980s.

Although Infante's group claimed to have demonstrated a dose-response relationship, critics argued that the exposure levels experienced by the Pliofilm workers were not known precisely enough to justify any such extrapolation. Suspicions about the study were exacerbated by the fact that the researchers were apparently urged by OSHA officials to publish their preliminary results quickly in order to support an upcoming rulemaking.

No More Knowledge, Less Policy Conflict

Our case studies also reveal instances where research findings reduced policy conflict without contributing much knowledge. This has been the case especially for negative epidemiological results. It is natural for such findings to be interpreted as an indication that the chemical under study does not cause cancer in humans. Yet our examination of the statistical power of cancer epidemiology shows that this impression is misleading. Still, relatively noninformative studies, which could not have detected the postulated risks, have influenced policy discussions.

Take for example NCI's large epidemiological study of formaldehyde, involving 27,000 workers and—initially—about 5,000 deaths. The investigators did a remarkable job of enlisting industrial support in an effort to obtain the best possible exposure information. Yet when all the dust had settled, the study revealed no clear link between formaldehyde and cancer.

When these results were released, many news agencies ran headlines—based on NCI's press release—suggesting that the study showed little evidence for concern about human cancer risk. Our analysis in Chapter 3 showed, however, that if the human risk estimates extrapolated from the CIIT rat data are true, they would not have been detected by even this relatively large and sophisticated cohort study. Indeed the study probably could not have detected risk levels comparable to the numerical thresholds of significant risk used by federal regulatory agencies.

Despite the fact that, properly understood, these results added little to relevant knowledge, our informal communications with participants in the formaldehyde controversy suggests that the NCI study may have reduced policy conflict. At least some of the participants now claim that humans are less sensitive to the carcinogenic action of formaldehyde than rats. While this may or may not be true, the NCI study simply did not illuminate this hypothesis, its policy impact notwithstanding.

No More Knowledge, No Effect on Policy Conflict

As a final example of a different sort, consider quantitative risk assessment. As it is currently practiced, we believe that this method has often provided little knowledge and also has done little to resolve policy conflict, despite the attention focused upon it.

The key assumptions made by agency risk assessors—no threshold in the dose-response function and linearity at low doses, use of cumulative lifetime exposure as the measure of dose, and a presumption that humans are as sensitive as the most sensitive animal species tested—were not clearly wrong in the case of either formaldehyde or benzene. Indeed, various theories and conjectures about carcinogenesis make these assumptions seem plausible to a substantial segment of the scientific community. The difficulty is that alternative technical assumptions are also plausible, have support among many scientists, and often lead to radically different risk estimates from those produced by federal agencies.

The range of risk estimates reported in Chapter 6 for benzene does not fully convey the range of opinion on this question. Some scientists, such as Jandl, are inclined to believe that the risk of cancer from exposure to low doses of benzene is zero. They remain unconvinced that any of the formal methods of risk assessment in widespread use are very informative. The risk estimates for formaldehyde exposure reported by CPSC and EPA also conceal huge scientific uncertainties. For example, what exactly should we assume about the dose-response function for the widespread, low, environmental exposures? OSHA's risk assessment made a more concerted effort to convey some of the major unknowns by highlighting how uncertain the results of models are in the face of the underlying uncertainty about mechanisms of carcinogenesis.

Perhaps because of these weaknesses, our case studies provided little evidence that numerical risk estimates resolved policy conflict. Consider, in particular, how the risk estimates for formaldehyde produced by CPSC were a focal point for criticism by industry and were ultimately found wanting by a federal appeals court. The range of risk estimates reported by OSHA was wide enough to be compatible with virtually any policy belief. EPA's risk numbers were generally ignored by the agency under Gorsuch and embraced under Ruckelshaus, although under Ruckelshaus EPA chose to ignore the large estimates of risk to the general population of formaldehyde in urban air since they had unsettling policy implications. Both in this case and in the benzene history, actors in the policy process tended to embrace the numbers when they supported their predetermined policy position and ignored or criticized the numbers when they led to contrary policy implications. We found few cases where numerical risk estimates changed regulators' opinions or drove policy decisions.

The Fundamental Role of Political Conflict

In summary, our case studies suggest that scientific research does not always create knowledge and, even when it does, the resulting knowledge does not necessarily reduce policy conflict. In part this is because direct, reliable knowledge about the risks of cancer at low doses is so difficult to obtain. But that is not the whole story. Differences in ideology and interest are both common and intense when it comes to controlling chemical carcinogens, and these factors can be expected to sustain policy conflict even in the presence of some clear technical results—assuming the stakes are high enough.

When policy conflict about a chemical arises primarily from differing opinions about how regulators should act in the face of uncertainty, it is possible that science—by reducing uncertainty—can diminish policy conflict. In other situations, however, we should expect increases in scientific knowledge to sharpen—or at least make explicit—the underlying political disagreements. By more clearly identifying winners and losers in chemical regulation, science can actually help activate conflicting interest groups and make it more difficult to resolve policy disagreements.

A clear example of knowledge about a toxic substance not resolving policy conflict is smoking. The fact that the mortality and morbidity effects of tobacco are known with some precision—much, much more precisely than for almost any other carcinogen—has done much to sharpen awareness of the economic importance of the industry and to foster debate about the proper scope of personal freedom in our society. The knowledge has not generated a policy consensus, although recent evidence of adverse health effects from passive smoking may prove to be more influential. Based on the tobacco experience, one should not be confident that adding any particular piece of knowledge about a widely used chemical carcinogen will necessarily lead to resolution of policy conflict.

• The Dangers of Overselling Science

We believe it is important to appreciate the limits of what science and scientists can do to resolve policy conflict because there are real dangers in making overly ambitious claims about the role of science in this area. When science is oversold, nonexperts, particularly interested citizens and politicians, tend to develop unrealistic expectations about what science can deliver. When it turns out that science cannot deliver on these expectations, public trust and confidence in science will suffer. The widespread publicity about the ineffectiveness of the National Cancer Institute's highly touted, multi-billion-dollar "war on cancer" is an excellent illustration of this phenomenon.[8]

The other danger of overselling science is that the accountable political actors will not face up to the value judgments that must be made in chemical regulation. Although regulators might prefer to pass the buck by hiding behind a cloak of quantitative risk assessment, it is important for a representative democracy to deliberate explicitly about the political aspects of chemical regulation. If regulators are not compelled to be explicit about the nature of their policy judgments, then it is unlikely that an informed public discussion of ethics and values will occur. Implicit and unexamined policy judgments are undesirable because they preclude accountability and complicate problem solving in the long run.

• The Contributions of Science to Regulation

At this point in the discussion, readers might be inclined to conclude that our position on chemical regulation is antiscientific. We intend no such inference. The advice provided by scientists and the knowledge generated by scientific research are critical to both the competency and legitimacy of public policy about chemical regulation. Even though science cannot always resolve or reduce policy conflict, it can make other important contributions. It is to help ensure that science can and does make these contributions that we urge a more searching and honest view of its concomitant limitations.

Discovering Unrecognized Chemical Hazards

First, science plays a vital role in legitimizing protective regulation by identifying hazardous chemical exposures that previously were not suspected to pose a risk of cancer to humans. In short, without science there is no basis for regulation. Illustrations from the case studies are numerous. The work by clinicians in Europe established that benzene is a human leukemogen. This knowledge was instrumental in triggering protective responses throughout the world. The work by toxicologists at CIIT was crucial in identifying formaldehyde as an animal carcinogen and a potential human carcinogen. This knowledge stimulated an explosion of epidemiological and toxicological research to better understand the possible risks to humans. It also triggered a variety of regulatory responses.

The irony is that this type of contribution is perhaps at least as likely to create or increase policy conflict as it is to reduce it. Raising suspicion about a chemical is bound to create pressure for regulation, and those with an economic interest in the chemical can be expected to resist regulation. Science is nonetheless making a beneficial contribution to the regulatory process when it creates policy conflict by calling attention to a previously unrecognized chemical hazard.

Ironically, when it comes to identifying hazards, our current scientific methods operate quite asymmetrically. Although science can raise concerns about a chemical's carcinogenic properties, it is not very helpful in proving that a truly innocuous substance poses no carcinogenic risk. Negative results from animal and human studies may place un upper bound on risk, but they do not prove complete safety. Similarly, once a chemical has been shown to cause cancer in animals or humans at high exposure levels, it is currently impossible to prove through science that low exposure levels are associated with no incremental risk. The cases of formaldehyde and benzene demonstrate that it is hard to imagine what scientific evidence could prove that small human exposures to these chemicals are not carcinogenic. Increasing knowledge is therefore likely to make the world seem to be an increasingly hazardous place—a process all too familiar to any regular newspaper reader.

Helping Regulators Set Priorities

A second role scientists can usefully play is in helping policy makers set regulatory priorities. Federal agencies have such limited administrative resources that they cannot possibly regulate the several hundred substances that have already been shown to produce cancer in humans or animals. Even though scientists cannot make defensible and exact quantitative statements about the low-dose risks of particular chemicals, they can offer informed judgments about the relative risks of various chemicals and mixtures at currently experienced doses. Regulators could benefit greatly from comparisons of chemicals in such terms.

Scientists might say, for example, that a lifetime of exposure to 10 ppm of benzene presents in their judgment a larger risk of cancer to a worker than a lifetime of exposure to 0.1 ppm of formaldehyde in the home. It is not necessary to understand precisely the risks posed by both chemicals in order to have a reasonable basis for such a conclusion. Even if scientists are not unanimous, a careful report on the distribution of their beliefs might be a very useful contribution to regulatory decision making.

In our case studies we found very little evidence that federal agencies solicit scientific advice of this sort in setting regulatory priorities. Instead, agencies tend to react to petitions from interest groups and then seek scientific advice on a case-by-case basis. Labor and environmental groups were the key priority-setting forces in the history of benzene and formaldehyde. We believe that if federal agencies sought and acted on more external scientific advice on the comparative risks of various chemicals, they would be able to expend their limited resources in a way that provided greater public health benefits.

Defining Better Measures of Exposure

The conventional practice of risk assessors and regulators is to define exposure in terms of either a TWA or a cumulative amount over a specified period of time. Relatively less attention has been given to the toxicological significance of the time pattern, such as the frequency and extent of peaks and valleys and the notion of intermittent exposure. Science can help regulators by informing them about what parameters of exposure are the most important to monitor and regulate.

Benzene and formaldehyde, it appears, may require a more sophisticated concept of dose if regulation is to be effective. We have already suggested that the failure of agencies to take these ideas seriously results in part from the fact that they disrupt traditional paradigms and assumptions. We nonetheless urge federal agencies to consider more seriously this kind of information; to do otherwise is to achieve bureaucratic ease at the heavy price of misconceived standards and regulations.

Providing Mechanistic Information

Finally, increased knowledge about the mechanisms of chemical carcinogenesis could give regulators more guidance about how to perform both interspecies and high-to-low dose extrapolations. During the next ten to twenty years, it is possible—some say likely—that we will have knowledge about the fundamental processes of carcinogenesis to help guide extrapolations.

The research by CIIT on the amount of formaldehyde delivered to DNA in the rat's respiratory lining is an illustration of the type of work that might help risk assessors. This work aims to illuminate how reducing the amount of formaldehyde inhaled by rats or people will affect the amount of formaldehyde that reaches target cells where cancer is initiated or promoted. Instead of just assuming that the delivered dose declines proportionately with the administered dose, risk assessors would have some empirical basis for estimating the actual relationship. As a result, extrapolation from high to low doses could be performed with a stronger scientific rationale.

Work on mechanisms can also help make interspecies extrapolation more tractable. Scientists at CIIT, for instance, are exploring how administered and delivered doses of formaldehyde are related in monkeys. The hope is that data from both rodents and monkeys will provide a stronger foundation for extrapolation of responses to humans than will data from rodents alone.

Such mechanistic research, like the experimental work by Irons on the responses of cells to intermittent benzene exposures, illustrates a relatively new and exciting approach to studying chemical carcinogenesis. Many scientists believe that the key to progress in this area is not more standard bioassays or traditional epidemiology, but more theoretical and empirical work on the mechanisms of cancer at the cellular level. Some scientists are also advocating molecular epidemiology that might be based on measuring certain biological markers (indicators) of exposure or disease in humans.

The trend in carcinogenesis research reflects a more general pattern in the maturation of scientific disciplines. As the limits of crude empiricism are recognized, scientists look for deeper understanding through disaggregation and new experimental techniques. Although it may take a long time to generate reliable mechanistic information for a large number of chemicals, this "new biology" should ultimately place public policy making on a stronger scientific footing.

Better Quantitative Risk Assessment

One area in which our case studies suggest that scientists have to do a better job is that of quantitative risk assessment. Federal agencies have come to place increasing emphasis on such methods in the regulatory process. These agencies then produce numbers that are used to justify decisions about what risks are deemed significant and to justify limitations on exposures or emissions. The Supreme Court's invalidation of OSHA's proposed benzene standard in 1980 has caused analysts at federal agencies to try to justify their agency's decisions by using such quantitative risk estimates.

Since risk estimates seem destined to play an increased role in the regulatory process, we believe it is important to devote more effort to doing that job well. The dominant practice in federal agencies is to produce a single risk number for each chemical based on a particular procedure developed by EPA's Carcinogen Assessment Group.[9] As we discussed in Chapter 6, the procedure is intended to produce a conservative, or "plausible upper-bound," estimate of risk based on a series of assumptions: use of data from the most sensitive animal species, inclusion of both benign and malignant tumors in animals, use of the multistage model for low-dose extrapolation, with constraints on its predictions so that the dose-response function is linear at low doses, and use of cumulative lifetime exposure as the measure of dose. The same assumptions are applied to each animal carcinogen. Where positive human data are available, the one-hit (linear) model is used to perform low-dose extrapolation of epidemiological findings.

In our view the CAG procedure represented a reasonable first step beyond the earlier practice of simply classifying chemicals as carcinogens or noncarcinogens. It is important to consider the magnitude of cancer risks, but unfortunately, the CAG procedure has major defects. It both conveys false precision and fails to incorporate all available scientific data and judgment. Risk assessors could take some specific new steps to make quantitative risk assessment more meaningful and honest. Some of these steps, which we describe below, are already being implemented by analysts at some federal agencies.

Improved Representation of Scientific Uncertainty

The single risk number often reported by federal agencies conceals enormous scientific uncertainty about chemical carcinogenesis. A more honest approach would be to report a range of risk estimates based on alternative sets of data and hypotheses. For example, risk estimates should be produced not just for the most sensitive animal species but also for other animal species that have been tested. Risk estimates based on alternative low-dose extrapolation models should also be reported, as OSHA did for formaldehyde. By producing such varied estimates, analysts would make clear to regulators and the public how little is known and why policy decisions must include judgments about the treatment of uncertainty.

One drawback of reporting numerical ranges is that we can never be sure that the range is wide enough to capture all of the biological and statistical uncertainties. In Chapter 6 we found that some of the assumptions used by CAG were not the most conservative imaginable. If one just sets extreme upper and lower bounds on the risk, then reporting the resulting range becomes quite unhelpful. The risk assessor will almost always find zero risk as a lower bound on low-dose risk and some quite large number as the "largest possible" upper bound. Yet such results convey almost nothing of what is known about the risks of the substance in question.

We believe that risk assessors should work with scientists to devise procedures for obtaining and conveying more information about scientific knowledge and beliefs concerning risks of various chemicals. Regulators need to know what possibilities are viewed as most likely and what alternatives are reasonably plausible in addition to the highly unlikely upper bounds. One way to do this would be to elicit from scientists their views about the plausible range of risk in the form of judgmental 80 percent probability or credibility intervals. The idea is to find upper and lower risk estimates that a scientist believes are 80 percent likely to include the true yet unknown risk. (The 80 percent figure is arbitrary—the precise value should be specified by each regulatory agency.) Since scientists can be expected to disagree about such intervals, risk assessors should elicit and report the judgments of a number of experts. EPA has already taken some preliminary steps toward implementing this type of approach to risk assessment.

In addition to reporting the interval within which risk is likely to fall, risk assessors should also try to elicit individual "best estimates" of risk from a number of working scientists.[10] This exercise will require those scientists to go beyond the available hard data and offer speculative forecasts of what is most likely to prove to be true when the uncertainty about chemical carcinogenesis is resolved.

A judgmental best estimate of risk might be especially useful as regulators set priorities. Two chemicals do not necessarily deserve equal rulemaking priority just because their upper-bound risk numbers are comparable, especially if the best estimate of risk is quite a bit larger for one of them. Although regulators might not—and we believe should not—base rulemaking decisions solely on best estimates of risk, this information could be a useful contribution to the priority setting process.

Some analysts might wonder why scientists should provide regulators with anything less than what decision theorists would call a complete judgmental probability distribution over cancer risk. Our suspicion is that an attempt to go beyond relatively simple probabilistic ranges will strain the willingness of cautious scientists to participate in the process. The additional information provided by the complete distribution might not be worth the difficulty and diminished intuitive plausibility associated with the more elaborate approach. In any case, the appropriate first step is to get some information about the true extent of scientific uncertainty along the lines suggested here or in some other way.

We recognize that there is likely to be significant resistance to such judgmental approaches. Most cancer researchers believe that there is a real external world out there and that their role in life is to discover that reality. The central mission of science is to search for truth; a theory, idea, or number is either true, false, or unknown. For many working scientists, the idea of judgmental estimates of cancer risk in the face of uncertainty is a confused or strained notion.

Ironically, scientists often behave in judgmental ways when they make professional decisions. (For example, in choosing what experiments to do, they consider subjectively the likelihood of various research strategies paying off.) The CIIT formaldehyde bioassay would never have been undertaken without the belief that there was a good chance that the study would have positive results—a good enough chance to make the major undertaking worthwhile. One can see the decisions that shape a scientist's entire research career as being based on a series of such estimates of the probabilities of various consequences of taking certain actions now. The problem is that such decision-theoretic thinking is not easily transferred from the process of resource allocation to consideration of the probabilistic nature of scientific truth.

A major task for risk and decision analysts, then, is to devise methods for eliciting scientific judgments and probability estimates that are feasible for use by federal agencies and also thoughtful enough to command the participation of working scientists.[11] These methods must be devised with the explicit understanding that scientists are not expected to agree necessarily about what estimates of excess cancer risk are most likely to prove true. The point is not to search for the one "true" estimate of uncertainty but rather to convey the variation in such estimates. The resulting range of scientific judgments must also be conveyed to regulators and to the public. Scientists should also be asked what research strategies are likely to help narrow the large ranges of uncertainty about cancer risk.

Incorporation of Mechanistic Information

Because of our belief in the value of mechanistic information, we feel that agencies should use such data to improve quantitative risk assessment.[12] Although today relatively little information exists about the mechanisms of chemical carcinogenesis, at least for benzene and formaldehyde, such data will, we hope, become increasingly available in the not too distant future.

The early indications are that federal agencies are reluctant to utilize mechanistic information. EPA's hesitant reaction to CIIT's delivered-dose data on formaldehyde is an example of this reluctance. It is hard to reconcile such information with current risk-assessment procedures; the data may not be perfectly reliable; and the data may often lead to less conservative risk estimates than would otherwise be produced.

Despite these problems, we urge agencies to use such data, at least as another approach to devising a range of risk estimates. If mechanistic information is ignored, scientists will be discouraged from working on mechanisms of carcinogenesis. We believe such investigations offer our best long-run hope for diminishing the current uncertainty about low-dose cancer risks.

Individual and Population Risk

Finally, risk assessors need to recognize that their efforts should be useful to regulators and others with a variety of value perspectives. The information they provide must be relevant both to those who are concerned about chemicals that impose large cancer risks on a small number of people and to those who are concerned about chemicals that impose small cancer risks on many people.

EPA's flipflop on formaldehyde under section 4(f) of the Toxic Substances Control Act (TSCA) illustrates why both kinds of information can be relevant. The EPA under Gorsuch chose not to trigger TSCA in the case of formaldehyde because it did not deem any individual risk to be sufficiently serious. Under Ruckelshaus the agency concurred with Gorsuch's value judgment about individual risk but argued that the population's exposure to formaldehyde was so "widespread" that a rulemaking investigation was appropriate. Although OSHA is often concerned primarily with controlling large individual risks to workers, EPA and CPSC are frequently concerned with regulating small individual risks that might add up to significant population risks. Hence, a risk-assessment report must address both aspects if it is to be fully informative.

▪ Expanding Risk Management Options

Using science more effectively to set priorities and to inform a more sophisticated approach to risk asssessment will not be sufficient to ameliorate all the difficulties of miscommunication and misunderstanding described in our cases. Nor will it be sufficient simply to encourage people to make more precise and modest claims for the role of scientific knowledge. Political incentives will always be there for executive irresponsibility and dishonesty about the basis for difficult choices and the risks of modern industrial life.

If we want the regulatory process to call forth and respond to a more sophisticated view of the available science, society must create a context in which the added informational complexity is worthwhile. In part for this reason, the legislative and administrative frameworks for dealing with chemical carcinogens need to be expanded to include a more diverse menu of risk-management options than exist now.

The more elaborate risk assessments we have called for will be undertaken only if they respond to the genuine needs of agencies. Regulators whose mandate includes few risk-management options have no use for complex risk assessments and thus will not be inclined to pay the bill for them. All they can do is to sort chemicals into a few categories for decision purposes. OSHA's generic cancer rule was designed to formalize such a simple sorting process. By enlarging the regulator's menu of decision options, Congress would create a need for a more elaborate sorting. This would allow for—and indeed foster—the use of more mechanistic information and scientific judgments.

An expanded set of risk-management options will make not only for better science, or the better use of science, but also for better policy. We need to learn to distinguish between those cases where a chemical has little social value (and hence can be severely restricted when we have only minimal evidence of risk) and those cases where the costs of inappropriate regulation would be substantial.

Efforts to create regulations that are not justified by the risk only divert resources from cases where regulation might do more good in terms of health protection. Overly simple rules that lead to extensive regulation also create the risk that relatively innocuous compounds will be assiduously pursued—only to result in the increased use of still more dangerous alternatives. The difficult cases are those where there are serious social and economic costs to regulation and also unknown but conceivably nontrivial health risks. We need a varied repertoire in order to tailor our responses to the details of the case at hand.

Our case studies reveal that legislation and court decisions often restrict the risk-management options available to regulators. OSHA, for example, is required to mandate the lowest feasible exposure levels for carcinogens in the workplace that can be achieved through engineering controls. EPA under section 112 of the Clean Air Act must set uniform national emission standards for airborne carcinogens at a level that protects the public health with an "ample margin of safety." These injunctions imply some flexibility, since the key terms are ambiguous and subject to interpretation. Neither agency, however, has the kind of discretion available to the CPSC, which can order labeling, set product safety standards, and promulgate bans.

Many authors have argued that Congress should allow regulators to consider various alternatives to strict command-and-control regulations, such as consumer or worker information, economic incentives through taxes or insurance, compensation to producers and victims of chemical exposure, and regional variation in regulatory programs. Economists in particular have argued that these alternatives may in many cases be more effective or less costly than command-and-control regulation.[13] Although we see merit in these arguments, we are offering an additional rationale for having more risk-management strategies.

▪ Proposals for Institutional Reform

Thus far we have advanced some of our own ideas about how science might be used more effectively in the regulatory process. In this section we describe and critique various other proposals for institutional reform that have been advanced to clarify or resolve conflicts about the regulation of chemical carcinogens. Experiments with some of these reforms were evident in the case studies of benzene and formaldehyde.

These proposals seem to fall into two categories: those that seek to resolve policy disputes by resolving scientific conflict and those that seek to bypass scientific conflict through political mechanisms. Although some of these reforms have merit, they all fail to address the central problems we have identified in the science-policy partnership: namely, the limits on scientific knowledge, the disjunctions between scientific and legal conceptualizations of the world, and the need for both science and values to be combined more explicitly in regulatory decision making.

Generic Rules and Uniform Guidelines

One of the most common suggestions of those who seek to decrease scientific conflict about carcinogen policy is to create strict generic rules for assessing chemical risks within each agency, and even to develop uniform guidelines for such assessments across all federal agencies. In the formaldehyde case study, we saw the influence of OSHA's generic cancer rule and the "cancer policy" guidelines of the Interagency Regulatory Liaison Group.[14] And in Chapter 1 we mentioned a 1983 report of the National Academy of Sciences that recommended a uniform policy for the production and use of risk assessments across federal agencies.[15]

The earliest cancer assessment guidelines and rules were intended to provide only qualitative determinations. They were to provide a simple yes or no answer to the question of whether compound X is a carcinogen. In the more recent and ambitious NAS formulation, the plan is to promulgate uniform guidelines for doing quantitative cancer risk assessment. In partial response to this NAS plan, EPA has in fact issued guidelines for quantitation.[16]

Although agencies have gone from qualitative to quantitative assessments, the underlying arguments for uniform guidelines are similar. Policy disputes about regulating chemical carcinogens are viewed as arising (in part) from the failure of federal agencies to use consistent methods for answering scientific issues, thereby allowing or even encouraging scientific disputes to continue. The presumption is that uniform assessment guidelines would reduce or eliminate policy conflict by purging the process of unnecessary, inappropriate, or dysfuntional scientific conflict.

Furthermore, it is argued that uniform rules make for a "government of laws not men." Guidelines let all parties know the rules of the game in advance and therefore strengthen the agency's hand in the litigation that all too frequently follows regulatory decisions. A predicted side benefit of uniform guidelines is faster and less costly rulemaking, since certain general issues (such as the existence or nonexistence of no-effect thresholds for carcinogens) would not be argued on a case-by-case basis.

Given the large number of analytical choices in estimating low-dose cancer risks, many types of uniform guidelines might be considered. If the guidelines are designed to be extremely conservative, that is, likely to overestimate actual risk, they will result in more pressure to regulate many low-level chemical exposures. Less conservative guidelines will generate fewer candidates for regulation. As we saw in Chapter 6, the analytic procedures used by federal agencies are based on a combination of very conservative guidelines.[17]

A fundamental problem with uniform guidelines—regardless of how conservative they are—is that they make it impossible for regulators or other interested parties to judge how conservative the final risk estimates are for a particular chemcial. This problem occurs because the same guideline (say, the use of toxicological data from the most sensitive species) is sure to create more conservative risk estimates for some chemicals than for others. When making a specific regulatory decision, regulators are then forced to accept the highly unpredictable conservatism embedded in the uniform risk assessment guidelines applied to the situation at hand. It becomes virtually impossible to achieve political accountability for the resulting policy judgments, especially since uniform guidelines will not produce the same degree of conservatism for each chemical. With such uniformity, it indeed becomes impossible to be equally conservative in each case.

Uniform guidelines also divert attention from the fact that the appropriate degree of conservatism to be used in risk assessment and risk management should be decided explicitly, and that doing so is ultimately a policy rather than a technical decision. Yet when the guidelines are drafted by "experts," the wrong impression is created about what types of choices are being made. As our cases show, regulators of different political persuasions often have different attitudes about how conservatively to act in the face of uncertainty about cancer risk, reflecting some of the divergent views in society at large, and this is as it should be. These are exactly the kinds of decisions for which elected officials and the public managers they appoint can and should be held accountable.

The 1983 NAS report was perhaps the most articulate and sophisticated statement in favor of uniform guidelines. Although we share many of the NAS committee's concerns about risk assessment, we do not believe that uniform risk assessment guidelines are steps in the right direction, any more than the earlier agency cancer policies were. Uniform rules and guidelines are likely—indeed are designed—to discourage the explicit expression of alternative beliefs and uncertainties that, as we argued previously, it is vital to encourage. Regulators should be presented with the full range of plausible scientific judgments about what the risks might be, at least in cases involving useful substances when it pays to make the rulemaking decision carefully. Only when rules or guidelines embody well-established *scientific knowledge* about cancer should they be accorded the presumptive status the NAS report proposes. And since carcinogenic processes are likely to be varied and complex, many uniform guidelines may well prove to be inaccurate and unsatisfactory as the findings of mechanistic research accumulate.

We take this position because we believe that one cannot and should not try to suppress scientific disagreements and uncertainties about an important chemical's potential carcinogenicity to humans. First, such attempts are quite likely to fail, as the case studies of formaldehyde and benzene indicate. Proponents of useful chemicals will demand that some forum (Congress, agencies, OMB, or the courts) be provided for a careful case-specific deliberation, notwithstanding the generic guideline. Second, and perhaps more important, such efforts are basically deceptive and miseducational. Trying to persuade citizens that risk estimates for all chemicals can be made on the basis of uniform guidelines will only lead them to misunderstand the full range of data and technical judgments that are involved in any regulatory decision. When scientists don't know much about cancer risk at low doses, making up some socially sanctioned number through an elaborate ritual only impairs our society's capacity to hold regulators accountable for their policy judgments.

The NAS committee appeared to have our view in mind when it wrote:

Guidelines very different from the kinds described could be designed to be devoid of risk assessment policy choices. They would state the scientifically plausible inference options for each risk assessment component without attempting to select or even suggest a preferred inference option. However, a risk assessment based on such guidelines (containing all the plausible options for perhaps 40 components) could result in such a wide range of risk estimates that the analysis would not be useful to a regulator or to the public.[18]

Our position nevertheless is that the full range of plausible scientific judgments should be reported, even if that might be less "useful" for resolving political conflict in the short run than a more definitive-sounding risk estimate.

Not only is it more honest, but the approach of reporting the range of risk numbers that scientists believe plausible, like our proposal for an 80 percent credibility range together with some measure of central tendency, is likely to be more beneficial in the long run. When actors in the regulatory process (including ordinary citizens) understand the true extent of scientific uncertainty, their expectations of science will be more realistic and the case for doing the critical mechanistic research will be strengthened. It is this research, we believe, that holds the promise for honestly reducing uncertainty about low-dose cancer risks.

Scientific Consensus Conferences

A second institutional device often recommended as a way to reduce scientific and hence policy conflict is the scientific consensus conference.[19] IARC performs this function on a regular basis for some chemicals. Committees of the NAS are also created on occasion to perform this service. Our case study of formaldehyde highlighted the activities at two ad hoc conferences: the Federal Panel on Formaldehyde and the Consensus Workshop on Formaldehyde. Our impression from observing regulatory practice at the federal level is that the scientific consensus approach is becoming more widely embraced to cope with disputes about chemical regulation.

We see two levels of ambition for such meetings and, implicitly, two slightly different theories that would govern their design and execution. The modest ambition is to achieve information exchange. The more lofty ambition is to actually achieve a consensus among participants about how to respond to the key questions posed by regulatory agencies. As we explain below, our view of the science-policy relationship is compatible only with the more modest ambition.

A sensible rationale for the modest ambition is that scientists working on a problem in different settings and from different disciplinary backgrounds will both contribute to and gain from a meeting with others working on related problems. Different scientific perspectives on a chemical can provide useful correctives, highlighting unexamined bias, wishful thinking, and new analytic methods or sources of data. Face-to-face communication can also speed the diffusion of new ideas, methods, and results—without the often lengthy time lag associated with scientific publication. As a result, scientific conferences can be expected to achieve a more rapid, dispassionate, and wide-ranging understanding of a chemical's toxicological properties than would otherwise be possible.

We believe that, properly run, scientific conferences serve a useful purpose by providing up-to-date information to individual scientists, interest groups, regulators, federal judges, chemical producers, and the public. By assembling evidence and identifying gaps in data, these conferences help chart the course of future research on a chemical's toxicological properties. For nonexperts these workshops can provide a comprehensive and readable summary of health-effects information.

For a conference to be of use to a regulatory agency, it is important that it be held relatively early in the agency's inquiry—preferably before it has published regulatory options or even a risk assessment document. Otherwise, the views of some individual scientists will have become manifest, and the positions of interest groups will have hardened. When strategic behavior has already begun, a conference is unlikely to influence the course of rulemaking. On the other hand, there must be enough data on a substance or issue to justify the time, travel, and expenses associated with a major conference.

The more lofty ambition for such meetings, the pursuit of consensus about answers to key questions posed by regulators, is from our perspective misguided. For such consensus is often sought in the hopes of reducing policy conflict precisely in those cases where it is least justified—that is, in the presence of real technical disagreements. In our opinion, the Consensus Workshop on Formaldehyde, which we described in Chapters 2 and 3, illustrated some of the dangers of this orientation. As the case study of formaldehyde reveals, there was substantial scientific disagreement about the carcinogenic properties of formaldehyde, and the Consensus Workshop did not even clarify—let alone resolve—these differences.

When consensus is defined as the goal, a superficial outcome can be expected. In their attempts to be cooperative, scientists may report only their centrist beliefs and avoid emphasizing uncertainties and sources of conflict. Cognitive psychologists have demonstrated that experts of all sorts have a general tendency to be overconfident in their judgments about uncertain quantities.[20] This tendency is often exacerbated by group dynamics. If "agreement" is an explicit goal of the conference, one can predict an accentuation of the tendency to downplay disagreement and uncertainty.

Our explication of the limits of science in this area makes clear that overt disagreements about the carcinogenic risks of a chemical at low doses do not necessarily mean either that anyone is making indefensible claims or behaving strategically. In our own scientific workshops on formaldehyde and benzene, we found that scientists were remarkably reluctant to be explicit about points of difference in scientific interpretation and judgment. Once we broke down this reluctance through extensive probing in an informal setting designed to legitimate disagreement, we found profound differences in views about the carcinogenic properties of both formaldehyde and benzene at low exposure levels. This richness of views did not emerge easily or spontaneously.

Even—or especially—when such conferences succeed in reporting an apparent consensus, we believe that the attempt to reduce regulatory controversy by trying to limit or ignore the technical—as opposed to political—sources of dispute is of dubious value. Well-intentioned scientists can all agree to agree, and in their search for agreement wind up accepting a superficial, unstable, misleading, or mistaken position. The Federal Panel on Formaldehyde's conclusion that formaldehyde is an animal carcinogen and "presumed" human carcinogen is an example of a unanimous yet superficial conclusion.

Consensus statements that paper over profound differences or unknowns foster a public misperception that more is known than in fact is known. Science is again oversold. In doing this, such meetings allow and encourage regulators to neglect important ethical and policy judgments about how to make decisions under uncertainty.

These issues are especially salient when conferences try to address the controversial task of quantifying cancer risk. For example, an attempt was made at the Consensus Workshop on Formaldehyde to have a risk estimation panel generate risk numbers based on inputs from various science panels. This working arrangement broke down when some observers objected that the numbers being computed by the risk estimation panel were not supported by the data submitted by the science panels. In the end the risk estimation panel offered no quantitative estimates.[21]

In our view this breakdown occurred in part because the results of the risk assessment were to be reported as point estimates rather than as ranges. Indeed, no attempt was made in the design of the meeting to record or to publish in the final document the disagreements among risk assessors that emerged. Nor was any attempt made to acknowledge the possibly central role of nonscientific, strategic values in the ultimately dysfunctional attempt to generate a single risk estimate.

Risk assessment should be designed to reflect the full range of scientific evidence and beliefs in quantitative risk estimates. To achieve this goal at conferences, we recommend that both practicing scientists and risk assessors be represented on panels. By involving scientists in the quantitative aspects of risk assessment, there is some assurance that the resulting numbers will reflect the data, the scientific conflicts, and the uncertainties. Likewise, risk assessors should be involved in the preparation of information on exposure and toxicity. This arrangement will allow science panels to report data and plausibility judgments that can be readily used by a risk-estimation panel. When scientists or risk assessors are not comfortable with the level of sophistication conveyed by quantification, they can insist upon a purely qualitative risk assessment.

Stricter Judicial Scrutiny

A third suggestion made by those who seek to limit policy conflict by operating on scientific conflict is that the judicial system should scrutinize how agencies use science.[22] According to this view the problem lies not so much in science but rather in the use of science by government. If only agencies could be forced to be "scientific," the argument goes, much policy conflict could be resolved.

In contrast to this view, our analysis of judicial review in Chapter 4 suggests some reasons to be pessimistic about the capacity of the courts—at least as currently designed—to "rationalize" administrative deliberations about potential chemical carcinogens.[23] The central problem is that many judges have rather limited understanding of the underlying scientific issues. They may also hold highly divergent and strong opinions about how key policy judgments in this area should be resolved by regulators. The conceptual doctrines that courts have developed (for example, significant risk) are a confusing mixture of scientific and policy considerations. Given the institutional isolation and limited technical competence of the federal judiciary, they cannot be expected to solve the dual problems of political and scientific conflict.

We do not mean to suggest that judicial review cannot play a constructive role in chemical controversies. The threat of lawsuits has clearly caused federal agencies to be more careful both in their procedures and their reasoning. On the other hand, this threat has also pushed some agencies in the direction of uniform, mechanical procedures with the hope that by limiting their own discretion they may find it easier to convince reviewing courts that they have been "fair" because "the numbers made me do it."

All things considered, we believe that judges should allow regulators substantial latitude in deciding which chemicals to regulate and how stringently to regulate them. Judges have no special expertise in the area of highly complex and uncertain science. Nor do they have any special claim to wisdom about how to act in the face of uncertainty or how to make value trade-offs between economics and health in the case of particular chemicals.

When Congress chose to delegate policy-making discretion to appointed officials of administrative agencies, a problem of political accountability was created. It is difficult to have citizens oversee the actions of these agencies. But intensive judicial second guessing transfers policy-making discretion to the judiciary and only aggravates the problem. Given the ambiguity of most of the basic statutes, judges should not thrust themselves into a central role in the process.[24] Instead, the normal constitutional mechanisms of executive responsibility and legislative oversight have to bear the burden of making democratic government work, even in this highly esoteric and difficult area.

Negotiated Rules

The institutional suggestions reviewed so far are aimed at somehow decreasing scientific conflict—or its effects. The last proposal we consider moves very far in the latter direction by, in a sense, ignoring the role of scientific disagreements altogether. Among those who are disappointed with the litigious nature of America's rulemaking process, there are some who hope that "negotiated" rules offer a viable solution.[25] The proposal is to get all the parties together to agree about the proper regulatory program.

Despite the failure of OSHA's benzene negotiations, we too see reasons to support the negotiation strategy. As an early paper produced by this project argued, this will be possible only under certain fairly restrictive conditions.[26] These include situations in which a small number of organized groups will incur most of the costs and the benefits of a regulation; in which credible representatives of these groups have the power to commit to, monitor, and enforce negotiated agreements; and in which a negotiated rule seems reasonably likely to make all parties better off (or at least not worse off) than they would be without a negotiated rule (when that calculation includes the costs they incur by participating in various alternative processes).

We have no precise sense as to how many controversies about potential carcinogens could meet these conditions, but we suspect that the number is small. This suspicion arises in part from our view that the costs of chemical regulations tend to be incurred more by members of society at large than by particular and identifiable producers. Moreover, chemcial exposures in the environment usually involve such a heterogeneous group of potential victims that designing appropriate citizen representation would be a formidable task. On the other hand, if participation is restricted, a negotiated rule may not prove to be a wise resolution of the problem since the unrepresented perspectives will tend to be disadvantaged.

Furthermore, regardless of how applicable or effective negotiated rulemakings might be, they do not obviate the need for a careful assessment of the range of evidence and judgments about the extent of cancer risk at various levels of exposure. Negotiators should understand the sources of technical disagreement about a chemical's risk of causing cancer in humans, even if this awareness complicates negotiations. In many cases presenting various scientists' beliefs about what is known, unknown, and suspected about a chemical's adverse effects could facilitate the negotiation process.

Advocates of this approach do not suggest, and we certainly do not approve of, negotiation in the form of, say, trading a particular interspecies scaling factor for a particular model of low-dose extrapolation. We are talking here about negotiation of policy, not science. Making cancer risk estimates through horse-trading would most assuredly not be a step in the right direction. Negotiated settlements should not only be *agreeable* but also—to the extent possible—based on responsible and explicit views about the science.

• Conclusion

The central message of this book is that actors in the regulatory process—regulators, scientists, interest groups, judges, journalists, and ordinary citizens—can benefit from a more precise and honest view of the ability of science and scientists to resolve disputes about chemical carcinogens. To shed light on this message, we believe it is useful to consider two polar positions on the role of science in the regulatory process.

One view holds that the key to satisfactory resolution of policy disputes about chemical carcinogens is to work toward achieving scientific consensus in the short run and to do more scientific research to reduce or resolve uncertainties in the long run. Since one of the fundamental sources of policy controversy is divergent values about how to act in the face of uncertainty, it seems plausible to predict that less uncertainty will foster less policy disagreement and more competent policy making. According to this view, the proper societal strategy is to emphasize the role of science and scientists as tools for conflict resolution.

A quite different view is that politics is and should be the master of influences on regulatory decisions about chemical carcinogens. The argument goes that science and scientists in this area are merely ammunition in a larger political struggle over conflicting values, interests, and sources of power. According to this view, there are no correct answers to questions about the regulation of chemical carcinogens, and scientific contributions are neither objective nor neutral. The implication for societal strategy in the United States is institutional reform to strengthen the democratic and participatory aspects of the regulatory process.

Between these polar viewpoints, we advance what might be called a "neoseparationist" view of the proper role of science in the regulatory process. Our position is not strictly separationist because we believe that it is impossible to completely separate scientific and political contributions to regulatory decision making.[27] The position is neoseparationist in that we call for a good-faith attempt by regulatory institutions to address separately and explicitly the extent of risks from chemical exposures and the acceptability of such risks.[28]

Neoseparationism implies that science and scientists have a modest yet important role to play in the regulatory process. The knowledge produced by science and by scientists' judgments provide essential guidance about regulatory choices: targeting neglected hazards, helping set priorities, and providing mechanistic information about the probable magnitude of low-dose risks. Science cannot prove that chemical exposures are "safe" and, at least in the short run, cannot provide reliable point estimates of low-dose chemical risks. In the years and decades ahead, the nation's investment in mechanistic research will probably provide a more informed basis for improved, but still imperfect, extrapolations of risks from rodents to humans and from high to low doses.

Neoseparationism also implies that science cannot answer the ultimate regulatory questions. Policy decisions must be made about the proper degree of conservatism in risk management, the proper societal trade-offs between public health and economic consequences, and the proper policy toward unequal distribution of cancer risks in the population. Only by recognizing the limited role of science as a resolver of conflict can these considerations be addressed explicitly and democratically. At the same time, modest expectations for science will prevent the public frustration and backlash against science that are likely if people hold inflated expectations about what it can deliver.

We believe that a precise and honest view about the role of science in chemical regulation will strengthen both science and democracy. Modest expectations in this area can be realized, and that means strengthened public confidence in science in the long run. Modest expectations for science also legitimize and foster explicit political discussion in our democracy about how to cope with chemical hazards.

▪ APPENDIX ▪ NOTES ▪ INDEX

▪ APPENDIX ▪ THE SCIENTIFIC CONFLICT MAPPING PROJECT

▪ *Meeting 1:* The Science-Policy Interface: Benzene and Formaldehyde
March 26, 1984

Chair: Dorothy Nelkin, Professor of Sociology, Cornell University

Participants: Roy Albert, Professor of Environmental Medicine, New York University Medical Center; Harvey Brooks, Professor of Applied Physics, Harvard University; Douglas Costle, Attorney, Wald, Harkrader, and Ross; J. Clarence Davies, Executive Vice President, Conservation Foundation; Paul Deisler, Vice President for Health, Safety, and Environment, Shell Oil Company; John Drake, Head of the Mutagenesis Section, National Institute of Environmental Health Sciences; Daniel Edwards, Director, Health and Safety Department, Oil, Chemical, and Atomic Workers Union; William Futrell, President, Environmental Law Institute; Maureen Henderson, Professor of Epidemiology and Medicine, University of Washington; Sheila Jasanoff, Senior Research Associate, Program on Science, Technology, and Society, Cornell University; Bruce Karrh, Corporate Medical Director, E. I. du Pont de Nemours and Company; James Mathis, Vice President of Science and Technology, Exxon Corporation; Lincoln Moses, Professor of Statistics, Stanford University; Henry Pitot, Professor of Oncology and Pathology, University of Wisconsin; Grover Wrenn, Principal, Environ, Inc.

▪ *Meeting 2:* Scientific Conflict about Formaldehyde
April 30, 1984

Chairs: Henry Pitot, Professor of Oncology and Pathology, University of Wisconsin; Lincoln Moses, Professor of Statistics, Stanford University

Participants: Harvey Brooks, Professor of Applied Physics, Harvard University; William Clark, Senior Scientist, Institute for Energy Analysis, Oak Ridge

Associated Universities; William DuMouchel, Associate Professor of Applied Mathematics, Massachusetts Institute of Technology; Joseph Fraumeni, Director of Epidemiology and Biostatistics Program, National Cancer Institute; Dale Hattis, Principal Research Associate, Center for Policy Alternatives, Massachusetts Institute of Technology; Sheila Jasanoff, Senior Research Associate, Program on Science, Technology, and Society, Cornell University; William Lowrance, Senior Fellow and Director of the Life Sciences and Public Policy Program, The Rockefeller University; Veronica Maher, Professor of Microbiology and Public Health, Michigan State University; Joyce McCann, Staff Scientist, Lawrence Berkeley Laboratory; Robert Miller, Chief, Clinical Epidemiology Branch, National Cancer Institute; Paul Nettesheim, Chief, Laboratory of Pulmonary Function and Toxicology, National Institute of Environmental Health Sciences; Maureen O'berg, Manager of Epidemiology Section, E. I. du Pont de Nemours Company; Howard Raiffa, Professor of Managerial Economics, Harvard University; Lawrence Susskind, Professor of Urban Studies and Planning, Massachusetts Institute of Technology; James Swenberg, Department Head, Biochemical Toxicology and Phenobiology, Chemical Industry Institute for Toxicology; William Thilly, Professor of Genetic Toxicology, Massachusetts Institute of Technology

- *Meeting 3:* Scientific Conflict about Benzene
  June 1, 1984

  Chair: John Drake, Head of the Mutagenesis Section, National Institute of Environmental Health Sciences

  Participants: John C. Bailar, Lecturer in Biostatistics, Harvard School of Public Health; William Clark, Senior Scientist, Institute for Energy Analysis, Oak Ridge Associated Universities; Philip Cole, Professor of Epidemiology, University of Alabama; Bernard Goldstein, Assistant Administrator for Research and Development, U.S. Environmental Protection Agency; David Hawkins, Senior Attorney, Natural Resources Defense Council; Richard Irons, Senior Scientist, Chemical Industry Institute of Toxicology; James Jandl, Professor of Medicine, Harvard Medical School; M. Gerald Ott, Research Leader in Epidemiology, Dow Chemical Company; Ellen Silbergeld, Chief Toxic Chemical Scientist, Environmental Defense Fund; William Thilly, Professor of Genetic Toxicology, Massachusetts Institute of Technology; Alice Whittemore, Professor of Family, Community, and Preventive Medicine, Stanford, University; James Wilson, Planning and Information Director, Environmental Policy Staff, Monsanto Company; Richard Wilson, Professor of Physics, Harvard University

▪ NOTES

▪ 1. Objectives and Methods

1. See William W. Lowrance, *Of Acceptable Risk* (Los Altos, Calif.: William Kaufman, 1976).
2. H. Seidman, M. S. Mushinski, S. K. Gelgvand, and E. Silberberg, "Probabilities of Eventually Developing or Dying of Cancer—United States, 1985," *CA—A Cancer Journal for Clinicians*, 35 (Jan./Feb. 1985): 36–56.
3. R. Doll and R. Peto, "The Causes of Cancer: Quantitative Estimates of Avoidable Risks of Cancer in United States Today," *Journal of the National Cancer Institute*, 66 (1981): 1191–1308. One opinion survey found that 80 percent of U. S. citizens (N = 1,488) felt that "'the chemicals we use" expose society to "more risk" today than existed twenty years ago. See *Risk in a Complex Society*, unpublished report by Louis Harris and Associates, 1980, p. 10.
4. See B. Fischhoff, P. Slovic, S. Lichtenstein, S. Read, and B. Combs, "How Safe Is Safe Enough? A Psychometric Study of Attitudes Towards Technological Risks and Benefits," *Policy Sciences*, 8 (1978): 127–152. The fear of cancer is reflected in recent surveys of the public's substantial willingness to pay money to prevent cancer. See, for example, M. W. Jones-Lee, M. Hammerton, and P. R. Phillips, "The Value of Safety: Results of a National Sample Survey," *Economic Journal*, 95 (Mar. 1985): 49–72.
5. John Cairns, *Cancer; Science and Society* (San Francisco: W. H. Freeman, 1978).
6. National Research Council, *Risk and Decision Making* (Washington, D.C.: National Academy Press, 1982), pp. 47–51.
7. On the general problem of science and policy, see Marc J. Roberts, Stephen R. Thomas, and Michael J. Dowling, "Mapping Scientific Disputes That Affect Public Policy Making," *Science, Technology, and Human Values*, 9 (Winter 1984): 112–122.
8. National Research Council, *Risk Assessment in the Federal Government: Managing the Process* (Washington, D.C.: National Academy Press, 1983).

9. See, for example, *Control of Carcinogens in the Environment,* Hearing before the Committee on Energy and Commerce, U.S. House of Representatives, 98th Cong., First Sess., Mar. 17, 1983; Paul F. Deisler, ed., *Reducing the Carcinogenic Risks in Industry* (New York: Marcel Dekker, 1984); Ronald Brickman, Sheila Jasanoff, and Thomas Ilgen, *Controlling Chemicals: The Politics of Regulation in Europe and the United States* (Ithaca: Cornell University Press, 1985); Mark E. Rushefsky, *Making Cancer Policy* (Albany: State University of New York Press, 1986).

- 2. Setting Regulatory Priorities

1. Formaldehyde Institute, *Formaldehyde: A Building Block of Our Society* (Scarsdale, N.Y.: Formaldehyde Institute, undated).
2. J. Walker, "Formaldehyde," *Kirk-Othmer Encyclopedia of Chemical Technology,* 10, 2nd ed. (1966), 77–99.
3. Formaldehyde Institute, *Formaldehyde.*
4. International Agency for Research of Cancer [IARC], *Monographs on the Evaluation of Carcinogenic Risk of Chemicals to Humans,* vol. 29, *Some Industrial Chemicals and Dyestuffs* (Geneva: World Health Organization, 1982), 353–356.
5. C. R. Mansfield et al., "Analysis of Formaldehyde in Tobacco Smoke by High Performance Liquid Chromatography," *Journal of Chromatography Science,* 15 (1977): 301–302.
6. L. E. Kane and Y. Alarie, "Sensory Irritation to Formaldehyde and Acrolein during Single Repeated Exposures in Mice," *American Industrial Hygiene Association Journal,* 38 (1977): 509–522.
7. W. P. Jordan, Jr., W. T. Sherman, and S. E. King, "Threshold Responses in Formaldehyde-Sensitive Subjects," *Journal of the American Academy of Dermatology,* 1 (1979): 44–48.
8. See *U.S. Code of Federal Regulations,* 29: 1910.1000 (b), Table Z–2. (hereafter cited as U.S. Code).
9. National Institute of Occupational Health and Safety [NIOSH], *Criteria for a Recommended Standard: Occupational Exposure to Formaldehyde* (Washington, D.C.: NIOSH, Dec. 1976), p. 2.
10. James Ramey, *FI Annual Report* (Scarsdale, N.Y.: Formaldehyde Institute, 1982), p. 2.
11. Nancy Harvey Stoerts, *Federal Response to Health Risks of Formaldehyde in Home Insulation, Mobile Homes, and Other Consumer Products,* Committee on Government Operations, U.S. House of Representatives, 97th Cong., 2nd Sess., May 18 and 19, 1982, p. 320. Estimate based on September 1981 survey of foam insulation contractors.
12. *Federal Register,* 44 (1979): 12080 (hereafter cited as *Fed. Reg.*).
13. U.S. Regulatory Council, "Statement on Regulation of Chemical Carcinogens," *Fed. Reg.,* 44 (1979): 60038.

14. This summary of the NAS findings is drawn from *Fed. Reg.*, 64 (1982): 14366–14367.

15. Ibid., pp. 14371, 14407.

16. *U.S. Code*, 15: 2056(b)(1).

17. *U.S. Code*, 15: 2052(a)(3).

18. *U.S. Code*, 15: 2058(c).

19. Southland Mower v. CPSC, 619 F.2d (5th Cir. 1980), p. 509.

20. Ibid., p. 789.

21. Aqua Slide 'N' Dive v. CPSC, 569 F.2d (5th Cir. 1978), pp. 842–843.

22. Forester v. CPSC, 599 F.2d (D.C. Cir. 1977), p. 788–789.

23. Richard A. Merrill, "CPSC Regulation of Cancer Risks in Consumer Products: 1972–1981," *Virginia Law Review*, 67 (Oct. 1981): 1264.

24. U.S. Consumer Product Safety Commission [CPSC], "Interim Policy and Procedure for Classifying, Evaluating, and Regulating Carcinogens in Consumer Products," *Fed. Reg.*, 43 (1978): 25658.

25. Dow Chemical, USA v. CPSC, 459 F. Supp. (W.D. La. 1978), p. 378.

26. *Fed. Reg.*, 45 (1980): 39434.

27. "Report of the Federal Panel on Formaldehyde," *Environmental Health Perspectives*, 43 (1982): 139.

28. *Fed. Reg.*, 46 (1981): 11188.

29. *Fed. Reg.*, 64 (1982): 14372.

30. Ibid., p. 14372.

31. For instance, see W. Kip Viscusi, *Regulating Consumer Product Safety* (Washington, D.C.: American Enterprise Institute for Public Policy Research, 1984).

32. For example, see "Product Safety Agency," *Congressional Quarterly Almanac* (1978): 525–528; and "CPSC Authorization," *Congressional Quarterly Almanac* (1981): 572–573.

33. I. J. Selikoff et al., *Carcinogenicity of Formaldehyde, Final Report* (New York: American Cancer Society, Feb. 25, 1981).

34. Statement adopted by the Board of Directors, American Cancer Society, New York City, Feb. 5, 1982.

35. Upton's letter is cited in Bette Hileman, "Formaldehyde: How Did EPA Develop Its Formaldehyde Cancer Policy," *Environmental Science and Technology*, 16 (1982): 544A.

36. See discussion of Bender's letter in Frederica Perera and Catherine Petito, "Formaldehyde: A Question of Cancer Policy?" *Science*, 216 (1982): 1287.

37. IARC, *Monographs on the Evaluation of Carcinogenic Risk*, 29: 20.

38. Hileman, "Formaldehyde," pp. 546A–547A.

39. The Higginson letter was subsequently quoted in Gulf South Insulation v. CPSC, 701 F.2d (5th Cir. 1983), pp. 1145–1146.

40. Ibid.

41. Gibson's letter is quoted in David J. Hanson, "Effects of Foam Insulation Ban Far Reaching," *Chemical and Engineering News*, Mar. 29, 1982, pp. 25–26.

42. Commissioner Stuart M. Statler voted against the ban because he believed that a product safety standard could adequately address the risk. *Fed. Reg.*, 47 (1982): 14365.

43. Marjorie Sun, "Formaldehyde Ban Is Overturned," *Science*, May 13, 1983, p. 699.

44. Hanson, "Effects of Foam Insulation Ban Far Reaching," pp. 34–37, esp. p. 35.

45. Gulf South Insulation v. CPSC, p. 1141.

46. Ibid., p. 1145.

47. Ibid., p. 1146.

48. Nicholas Ashford, C. William Ryan, and Charles C. Caldert, "Law and Science Policy in Federal Regulation of Formaldehyde," *Science*, 222 (1983): 894, 899–900.

49. Devra Lee Davis, "The Shotgun Wedding of Science and Law: Risk Assessment and Judicial Review," *Columbia Journal of Environmental Law*, 10 (1985): 67–109, esp. p. 85.

50. American Industrial Health Council, *Significant Developments Regarding Government Cancer Risk Assessment Methodology* (Washington, D.C.: American Industrial Health Council, 1983), pp. 3–7.

51. Richard Merrill, "The Legal System's Response to Scientific Uncertainty: The Role of Judicial Review," *Fundamental and Applied Toxicology*, 4 (1984): 5418, 5424–5425.

52. See *Fed. Reg.*, 48 (1983): 57478–57479.

53. *U.S. Code*, 29: 655(b)(5).

54. Industrial Union Dept. v. American Petroleum Institute, 448 U.S. 607 (1980).

55. American Textile Manufacturers Institute v. Donovan, 452 U.S. 490 (1981).

56. See *Fed. Reg.*, 42 (1977): 5148 (proposed generic cancer policy); and *Fed. Reg.*, 45 (1980): 5002 (final generic cancer policy).

57. *Fed. Reg.*, 46 (1981): 4889 (Bingham amends the generic standard to conform to the Supreme Court's ruling in the benzene case).

58. D. Hattis G. Mitchell, J. McCleary-Jones, and N. Gorelick, *Control of Occupational Exposures to Formaldehyde: A Case Study of Methodology for Assessing the Health and Economic Impacts of OSHA Health Standards* (Cambridge, Mass.: Center for Policy Alternatives, M.I.T., 1981).

59. See Joel R. Bender and Linda S. Mullin, *Criticisms of Health Aspects of Ashford Document*, mimeo (Wilmington, Del.: du Pont, May 27, 1981); and OSHA, *Preliminary Comments on Shortcomings of Ashford's Arguments for Further Regulation of Formaldehyde, and Observations as to What, If Anything, OSHA Should Do with Ashford's Study*, mimeo (Washington, D.C.: OSHA, May 28, 1981).

60. This account of the episode is based on Marjorie Sun, "A Firing over Formaldehyde," *Science*, 213 (1981); p. 630–631.

61. Ibid., p. 630.

62. *U.S. Code*, 29: 655(c).
63. Letter from Thorne Auchter, OSHA Administrator, to Howard Young, UAW, Jan. 29, 1982, mimeo.
64. United Auto Workers v. Donovan, U.S. District Court for the District of Columbia, Civil Action no. 82–2401, July 2, 1984, mimeo.
65. "Report on the Consensus Conference on Formaldehyde," *Environmental Health Perspectives*, 58 (Dec. 1984): 323–381.
66. UAW v. Donovan, p. 15.
67. Cathy Trost, "OSHA Chief's Stock Holdings in Blind Trust Prompt Conflict-of-Interest Criticism by Unions," *Wall Street Journal*, Apr. 17, 1985, p. 36.
68. *Fed. Reg.*, 50 (Jan. 11, 1985): 1547.
69. Letter from Robert A. Rowland, OSHA Administrator, to Franklin E. Mirer, UAW, Jan. 7, 1985, mimeo.
70. Dry Color Mfrs. Ass'n v. Dept. of Labor, 486 F.2d (3rd Cir. 1974), p. 98.
71. Public Citizen Health Research Group et al. v. Auchter, 702 F.2d (D.C. Cir. 1983), pp. 1150, 1156.
72. "OSHA Is Avoiding Regulatory Action through Risk Assessment, Mirer Charges," *Occupational Safety and Health Reporter*, Bureau of National Affairs (BNA), Jan. 17, 1985, p. 603.
73. "Memo Indicates OSHA Decided against ETS before Receiving Comments, Teamsters Charge," *Occupational Safety and Health Reporter* (BNA), Feb. 21, 1985, p. 731.
74. "UAW Charges That Formaldehyde Hearing Is 'Delaying Tactic' on Part of OSHA," *Occupational Safety and Health Reporter* (BNA), Feb. 21, 1985, pp. 731–732.
75. *Fed. Reg.*, 50 (1985): 15179–15184.
76. "Court Rejects OSHA's Move for Dismissal, Calls for 'Appropriate' Action by October," *Chemical Regulation Reporter* (BNA), June 14, 1985, p. 302.
77. Senate Report No. 94–698, reprinted in *U.S. Code Congressional and Administrative News*, 1976, p. 4491.
78. *U.S. Code*, 2603(f).
79. Nicholas A. Ashford, C. William Ryan, and Charles C. Caldert, "A Hard Look at Federal Regulation of Formaldehyde: A Departure from Reasoned Decisionmaking," *Harvard Environmental Law Review*, 7 (1983): 299.
80. The ensuing account of the Gorsuch administration's handling of formaldehyde is based on the testimony of Deputy Administrator John W. Hernandez, Jr., *Environmental Protection Agency: Private Meetings and Water Protection Programs*, U.S. House of Representatives, Subcommittee on Environment, Energy, and Natural Resources, 97th Cong., 1st sess., Oct. 21, 1981, pp. 14–22.
81. Ross Sandler, "Law: EPA's Secret 'Science Courts,'" *Environment*, 24 (Jan./Feb. 1982): 57.
82. Mark E. Rushefsky, "The Misuse of Science in Governmental Decision-

making," *Science, Technology, and Human Values,* 9 (Summer 1984): 47–59.

83. *Review of the Scientific Basis of the Environmental Protection Agency's Carcinogenic Risk Assessment of Formaldehyde,* report by Committee on Science and Technology, U.S. House of Representatives, 98th Cong., 1st Sess., 1983, p. 21.

84. Ibid., p. 22.

85. *Fed. Reg.,* 48 (1983): 52507–52508.

86. *Fed. Reg.,* 49 (1984): 21870, 21891.

87. For example, see E. D. Acheson et al., "Formaldehyde in the British Chemical Industry," *Lancet,* Mar. 17, 1984; pp. 611–616.

88. EPA reopened the 4(f) issue because of "public controversy" about the original decision. *Fed. Reg.,* 48 (Nov. 18, 1983): 52507–52508. Also see Marjorie Sun, "EPA May Be Redefining Toxic Substances," *Science,* 214 (1981): 525–526.

89. Michael Wines, "Scandals at EPA May Have Done In Reagan's Move to Ease Cancer Controls," *National Journal,* June 18, 1983, pp. 1264–1269.

90. "Science Advisory Board Asked to Review EPA Assessment of Risks Posed by Substance," *Chemical Regulation Reporter* (BNA), June 7, 1985: 283–284.

- 3. Interpreting the Scientific Evidence on Formaldehyde and Cancer

1. F. Watanabe, T. Matsunaga, T. Soejima, and Y. Iwata, "Study of the Carcinogenicity of Aldehyde. First Report: Experimentally Produced Rat Carcinomas by Repeated Injections of Aqueous Solution of Formaldehyde." *Gann,* 45 (1954): 451–452. A. W. Horton, R. Tye, and K. L. Stemmer, "Experimental Carcinogenesis of the Lung: Inhalation of Gaseous Formaldehyde or an Aerosol of Coal Tar by C&H Mice," *Journal of the National Cancer Institute,* 30 (1963): 31–43. H. S. Rosenkrantz, "Formaldehyde as a Possible Carcinogen," *Bulletin of Environmental Contamination and Toxicology,* 8 (1972): 242–244. P. Muller, G. Raabe, and D. Schumann, "Leukoplakia Induced by Repeated Deposition of Formalin in Rabbit Oral Mucosa: Long Term Experiments with a New Oral Tank," *Experimental Pathology,* 16 (1978): 36–42.

2. N. C. Morin and H. Kubinski, "Potential Toxicity of Materials Used for Home Insulation," *Ecotoxicology and Environmental Safety,* 2 (1978): 133–141.

3. W. D. Kerns, K. L. Pavkov, D. J. Donofrio, E. J. Gralla, and J. A. Swenberg,"Carcinogenicity of Formaldehyde in Rats and Mice after Long-term Inhalation Exposure," *Cancer Research,* 43 (1983): 4382–4392.

4. R. E. Albert, A. R. Sellakumar, S. Laskin, M. Kuschner, N. Nelson, and C. A. Snyder, "Gaseous Formaldehyde and Hydrogen Chloride Induction of Nasal Cancer in the Rat," *Journal of the National Cancer Institute,* 68 (1982): 597–603.

5. Kerns et al., "Carcinogenicity of Formaldehyde in Rats and Mice," p. 4387.

6. Brief of Petitioners, Formaldehyde Institute v. CPSC, 5th Circuit Court of Appeals, Case no. 82–4135, Sept. 30, 1982, p. 30 (hereafter cited as FI Brief).

7. D. G. Hoel, N. L. Kaplan, and M. W. Anderson, "Implication of Non-linear Kinetics on Risk Estimation in Carcinogenesis," *Science*, 219 (1983): 1032–1037.

8. P. J. Gehring, P. G. Watanabe, and C. N. Park, "Resolution of Dose-Response Toxicity Data for Chemicals Requiring Metabolic Activation: Example—Vinyl Chloride," *Toxicology and Applied Pharmacology*, 44 (1978): 581–591; C. Maltoni and G. Lefemine, "Carcinogenicity Assays of Vinyl Chloride: Current Results," *Annals of the New York Academy of Science*, 246 (1975): 195–224.

9. Joel B. Schwartz, Christine R. Riddiourgh, and Samuel S. Epstein, "Analysis of Carcinogenesis Dose-Response Relations with Dichotomous Data," *Teratogenesis, Carcinogenesis, and Mutagenesis*, 2 (1982): 179–204.

10. F. Stenback, R. Peto, and P. Shubik, "Initiation and Promotion at Different Ages and Doses in 2200 Mice III Linear Extrapolation from High Doses May Underestimate Tumor Risks," *British Journal of Cancer*, 44 (1981): 24–34.

11. J. Bailar, E. Crouch, R. Shaikh, and D. Spiegelman, "One-Hit Models of Carcinogenesis: Conservative or Not?" unpublished manuscript, 1986.

12. N. A. Littlefield, J. H. Farmer, D. W. Gaylor, and W. G. Sheldon, "Effects of Dose and Time in a Long-term, Low-dose Carcinogenic study," *Journal of Environmental Pathology and Toxicology*, 3 (1980): 17–34.

13. S. L. Graham, K. J. Davis, W. H. Hansen, and C. H. Graham, "Effects of Prolonged Ethylene Thiourea Ingestion on the Thyroid of the Rat," *Food and Cosmetic Toxicology*, 13 (1975): 493–499.

14. For a discussion of this hypothesis, see U.S. Office of Science and Technology Policy, "Chemical Carcinogens: A Review and Its Associated Principles," *Fed. Reg.*, 50 (1985): 10403–10410.

15. C. J. Shellabarger, V. P. Bond, E. P. Cronkite, and G. E. Aponte, "Relationship of Dose of Total-Body ^{60}C Radiation to Incidence of Mammary Neoplasia in Female Rats," in *Radiation-Induced Cancer* (Vienna: International Atomic Energy Agency, (1969), pp. 161–172; A. C. Upton, R. C. Allen, R. C. Brown, N. K. Clapp, J. W. Conklin, Jr., L. J. Serrano, R. L. Tyndall, and H. E. Walburg, Jr., "Quantitative Experimental Study of Low-Level Radiation Carcinogenesis," ibid., pp. 425–438.

16. Littlefield et al., "Effects of Dose and Time."

17. H. E. Walburg, "Experimental Radiation Carcinogenesis," *Advances in Radiation Biology*, 4 (1974): 210–245.

18. R. D. Evans, A. T. Keane, R. J. Kolenkow, W. R. Neal, and M. M.

Shanahan, *Delayed Effects of Bone-Seeking Radionuclides* (Salt Lake City: University of Utah Press, 1969), pp. 157–194.

19. D. W. Gaylor, "The ED Study: Summary and Conclusions," *Environmental Pathology and Toxicology*, 3 (1980): 179–183.

20. J. A. Swenberg, E. A. Gross, J. Martin, and J. A. Popp, "Mechanisms of Formaldehyde Toxicity," in *Formaldehyde Toxicity*, ed. J. E. Gibson, (Washington, D.C.: Hemisphere Publishing, 1983), pp. 132–137.

21. H. Heck, T. Y. Chin, and M. Schmitz, "Distribution of 14C Formaldehyde in Rats after Inhalation Exposure," in Gibson, *Formaldehyde Toxicity*, pp. 26–37.

22. M. C. Casanova-Schmitz and H. Heck, "Effects of Formaldehyde Exposure on the Extractability of DNA from Proteins in the Rat Nasal Mucosa," *Toxicology and Applied Pharmacology*, 70 (1983): 121–132.

23. M. Casanova-Schmitz, T. B. Starr, and H. Heck, "Differentiation between Metabolic Incorporation and Covalent Binding in the Labeling of Macromolecules in the Rat Nasal Mucosa and Bone Marrow by Inhaled [^{14}C] – and [^{3}H] Formaldehyde," *Toxicology and Applied Pharmacology*, 76 (1984): 26–44.

24. K. T. Morgan, D. L. Patterson, and E. A. Gross, "Formaldehyde and the Nasal Mucociliary Apparatus," in *Formaldehyde: Toxicology, Epidemiology and Mechanisms*, ed. J. J. Clary, J. E. Gibson, and R. S. Waritz (New York: Marcel Dekker, 1983), pp. 193–209.

25. T. Dahlman and J. Rhodin, "Effects of Exposure to Lung-Irritating Gas on Transport of Secretion and Fibrillation Frequency in Rat Trachea," *Nordisk Hygienisk Tidskrist*, 37 (1956): 82–90.

26. T. Y. Chin and H. D. Heck, "Disposition of 14C Formaldehyde in Fischer-344 Rats Following Inhalation Exposure" (abstract), *Toxicologist*, 1 (1981): 78.

27. Paul Nettesheim, 1984, personal communication.

28. Swenberg et al., "Mechanisms of Formaldehyde Toxicity," in Gibson, *Formaldehyde Toxicity*, p. 146.

29. European Chemical Industry Ecology and Toxicology Center [ECETOC], *The Mutagenic and Carcinogenic Potential of Formaldehyde*, Technical Report no. 2 (Brussels: ECETOC, 1981), p. 23.

30. E. Farber, "Chemical Carcinogenesis: A Biologic Perspective," *American Journal of Pathology*, 106 (1982): 272–296.

31. D. Hattis, G. Mitchell, J. McCleary-Jones, and N. Gorelick, *Control of Occupational Exposures to Formaldehyde: A Case Study of Methodology for Assessing the Health and Economic Impacts of OSHA Health Standards* (Cambridge, Mass.: Center for Policy Alternatives, M.I.T., 1981).

32. Swenberg et al., "Mechanisms of Formaldehyde Toxicity," in Gibson, *Formaldehyde Toxicity*, pp. 132–137.

33. ECETOC, *Mutagenic and Carcinogenic Potential of Formaldehyde*, pp. 23–24.

34. Kerns et al., "Carcinogenicity of Formaldehyde in Rats and Mice."

35. G. M. Rusch, J. J. Clary, W. E. Rinehart, and H. F. A. Bolte, "26-Week

Inhalation Toxicity Study with Formaldehyde in the Monkey, Rat, and Hamster," *Toxicology and Applied Pharmacology*, 68 (1983): 329–343.

36. T. R. Birdwell and L. J. Cole, *Early Alveolar Cell Mitotic Activity and Pulmonary Tumor Incidence in Urethane Treated X-Irradiated Mice*, Report USNRDL-TR-68-51 (Washington, D.C.: U.S. Radiological Defense Laboratory, 1968), pp. 1–11.

37. M. C. Henry and C. D. Port, "Effect of Anesthetic Agent on Lung Tumor Induction in Hamsters Given Benzo[a]-pyrene-Ferric Oxide," *Journal of the National Cancer Institute*, 61 (1978): 1221.

38. P. Nettesheim, D. D. Topping, and R. Jamasbi, "Host and Environmental Factors Enhancing Carcinogenesis in the Respiratory Tract," *Annual Review of Pharmacology and Toxicology*, 21 (1981): 133.

39. W. E. Dalbey, "Formaldehyde and Tumors in Hamster Respiratory Tract," *Toxicology*, 24 (1982): 9–14.

40. R. E. Albert, A. R. Sellakumar, S. Laskin, M. Kuschner, N. Nelson, and C. A. Snyder, "Gaseous Formaldehyde and Hydrogen Chloride Induction of Nasal Cancer in the Rat," *Journal of the National Cancer Institute*, 68 (1982): 597–603.

41. Kerns et al., "Carcinogenicity of Formaldehyde in Rats and Mice," p. 4387.

42. See, for example, OSHA, "Occupational Exposure to Formaldehyde," *Fed. Reg.*, 50 (1985): 50450.

43. R. A. Squire and L. L. Cameron, "An Analysis of Potential Carcinogen Risk for Formaldehyde," *Regulatory Toxicology and Pharmacology*, 4 (1984): 107–129.

44. Environmental Protection Agency, "Formaldehyde: Determination of Significant Risk," *Fed. Reg.*, 49 (1984): 21874.

45. Kerns et al., "Carcinogenicity of Formaldehyde in Rats and Mice."

46. OSHA, *Fed. Reg.*, 50 (1985): 50450.

47. FI Brief, p. 3.

48. National Research Council Committee on Aldehydes, *Formaldehyde and Other Aldehydes* (Washington, D.C.: National Academy Press, 1981).

49. Clary, Gibson, and Waritz, "Introduction," in *Formaldehyde: Toxicology, Epidemiology, and Mechanisms*, p. x.

50. OSHA, "Identification, Classification, and Regulation of Potential Occupational Carcinogens," *Fed. Reg.*, 45 (1980): 5129 (quoting Paul Kotin's testimony).

51. Ibid., p. 5130 (OSHA statement).

52. Ibid., p. 5130 (quoting David Rall's testimony).

53. Laura Green and Angela Boggs, "About Endogenous Formaldehyde," unpublished manuscript, 1988.

54. Letters to the Editor, *Toxicology and Applied Pharmacology*, 77 (1985): 363–368.

55. M. S. Cohn, F. J. DiCarlo, A. Turturro, and A. G. Ulsamer, ibid., pp. 363–364.

56. M. Casanova-Schmitz, T. B. Starr, and H. Heck, ibid., p. 365.

57. Cohn et al., ibid., p. 364.

58. Casanova-Schmitz et al., ibid., p. 367.

59. Swenberg et al., "Mechanisms of Formaldehyde Toxicity."

60. IARC, *Monographs on the Evaluation of Carcinogenic Risk of Chemicals to Humans*, 19 (Geneva: WHO, 1979), 377–438.

61. C. Maltoni, G. Lefemine, A. Ciliberti, G. Colti, and D. Cerretti, "Carcinogenicity Bioassays of Vinylchloride Monomer: A Model of Risk Assessment on an Experimental Basis," *Environmental Health Perspectives*, 41 (1981): 3–29.

62. J. L. Egle, Jr., "Retention of Inhaled Formaldehyde, Propionaldehyde, and Acrolein in the Dog," *Archives of Environmental Health*, 25 (1972): 119–124.

63. Watanabe et al., "Study of the Carcinogenicity of Aldehyde."

64. Muller et al., "Leukoplakia Induced by Repeated Deposition of Formalin."

65. R. G. Croy, J. M. Essigman, and G. N. Wogan, "Identification of the Principal Aflatoxin B_1-DNA Adduct Formed *In Vitro* in Rat Liver," *Proceedings of the National Academy of Sciences (USA)*, 15 (1978): 1745–1749.

66. "The Report on the Consensus Conference on Formaldehyde." *Environmental Health Perspectives*, 58 (Dec. 1984).

67. Maureen O'berg, 1984, personal communication.

68. E. D. Acheson, M. J. Gardner, B. Pannett, H. R. Barnes, C. Osmond, and C. P. Taylor, "Formaldehyde in the British Chemical Industry," *Lancet*, Mar. 17, 1984, pp. 611–616.

69. See "Report on the Consensus Conference on Formaldehyde," pp. 334–340.

70. T. Watanabe and D. M. Aviado, "Functional and Biochemical Effects on the Lung Following Inhalation of Cigarette Smoke and Constituents," *Toxicology and Applied Pharmacology*, 30 (1974): 201–209.

71. Horton et al., "Experimental Carcinogenesis of the Lung."

72. Surgeon General's Report, Department of Health, Education, and Welfare, *The Health Consequences of Smoking* (Washington, D.C.: U.S. Government Printing Office, 1972).

73. J. Higginson, Letter to Nancy Harvey Stoerts, U.S. Consumer Product Safety Commission, Feb. 12, 1982, mimeo.

74. "Report of the Federal Panel on Formaldehyde," *Environmental Health Perspectives*, 43 (1982): 139–168.

75. Acheson et al., "Formaldehyde in the British Chemical Industry."

76. Ibid.

77. Higginson, Letter to Stoerts, Feb. 12, 1982.

78. G. T. Ulitsky, S. L. Shalat, K. Riccardi, and N. J. Vianna, "Epidemiologic Patterns of Nasal Cancer in New York State," *Journal of Occupational Medicine*, 23 (Sept. 1981): 632–634.

79. J. H. Olsen, S. P. Jensen, M. Hink, K. Fawbo, N. O. Breumo, and O. M. Jensen, "Occupational Formaldehyde Exposure and Increased Nasal Cancer Risk in Man," *International Journal of Cancer*, 34 (1984): 639–644.

80. H. Heck, T. Y. Chin, and M. C. Schmitz, "Distribution of [^{14}C] Formaldehyde in Rats after Inhalation Exposure," in Gibson, *Formaldehyde Toxicity*, pp. 26–37.

81. See, generally, "Report on the Consensus Conference on Formaldehyde," pp. 346–348.

82. Ibid., p. 338.

83. Ibid.

84. J. M. Harrington and E. Oakes, "Mortality Study of British Pathologists, 1974–1980," unpublished manuscript.

85. IARC *Monographs on the Evaluation of Carcinogenic Risk*, 29 (1982): 375.

86. John A. Todhunter, Memo to Ann Gorsuch, 1982.

87. FI Brief, p. 4.

88. F. Perera and C. Petito, "Formaldehyde: A Question of Cancer Policy?" *Science*, 216 (1982): 1285–1291.

89. Higginson, Letter to Stoerts, Feb. 12, 1982.

90. Acheson et al., "Formaldehyde in the British Chemical Industry."

91. Ibid.

92. Editorial, "Formaldehyde and Cancer," *Lancet*, July 2, 1983, p. 26.

93. A. Blair et al., "Mortality among Industrial Workers Exposed to Formaldehyde," *Journal of the National Cancer Institute*, 76 (1986): 1071–1084.

94. I. A. Rapoport, "Carboxyl Compounds and the Chemical Mechanisms of Mutation," *Doklady Academii Nauk SSSR*, 54 (1946): 65–67; and W. D. Kaplan, "Formaldehyde as a Mutagen in Drosophila," *Science*, 108 (1948): 43.

95. C. Auerbach, M. Moutschen-Dahmen, and J. Moutschen, "Genetic and Cytogenetical Effects of Formaldehyde and Related Compounds," *Mutation Research*, 39 (1977): 317–362.

96. Ibid.; also C. J. Boreiko and D. Ragan, "Formaldehyde Effects in the C3H/10T1/2 Cell Transformation Assay," in *Proceedings of the Third Annual CIIT Conference: Formaldehyde Toxicity* (Research Triangle Park, N.C.: Chemical Industry Institute of Toxicology, 1982).

97. "Report on the Consensus Conference on Formaldehyde," p. 342.

98. Y. Sasaki and R. Endo, "Mutagenicity of Aldehydes in Salmonella" (Abstract no. 27), *Mutation Research*, 54 (1978): 251–252.

99. "Report on the Consensus Conference on Formaldehyde," p. 342.

100. OSHA, "Identification, Classification, and Regulation of Potential Occupational Carcinogens," *Fed. Reg.*, 45 (1980): 5160.

101. Ibid., p. 5173.

102. Ibid., p. 5171 (quoting L. Golberg).

103. "Report on the Consensus Conference on Formaldehyde," p. 342.

- 4. The Problem of Setting Standards

1. International Agency for Research of Cancer [IARC], *Monographs on the Evaluation of Carcinogenic Risk of Chemicals to Humans,* 29, (Geneva: World Health Organization, 1982), 95–96.
2. "Proposed OSHA Benzene Rule," *Fed. Reg.,* 50 (Dec. 10, 1985): 50540.
3. IARC, *Monographs on the Evaluation of Carcinogenic Risk,* 29 p. 101.
4. The ensuing account of OSHA's creation is based on two sources: Steven Kelman, "Occupational Safety and Health Administration," in *The Politics of Regulation,* ed. James Q. Wilson (New York: Basic Books, 1980), pp. 238–243; and John Mendeloff, *Regulating Safety: An Economic and Political Analysis of Occupational Safety and Health Policy* (Cambridge, Mass.: MIT Press, 1980), pp. 15–23.
5. Business lobbyists did win some concessions of independence in the enforcement process. See *Congressional Quarterly Almanac* (1970): 675–682.
6. *U.S. Code,* 29: 652(8).
7. See Vincent C. Baird, "IUD v. API: Limiting OSHA's Authority to Regulate Workplace Carcinogens under the Occupational Safety and Health Act," *Environmental Affairs,* 9 (1981): 651–652.
8. *U.S. Code,* 29, 655(b)(5).
9. The original Daniels bill was H.R. 16785, 91st Cong., 2nd Sess. (1970). The House Committee on Education and Labor reported an amended version of the Daniels bill containing the quoted passage. See House of Representatives (HR) Report no. 91–1291 (1970), p. 4; also *Legislative History of the Occupational Safety and Health Act of 1970,* Committee Print (Washington, D.C.: U.S. Government Printing Office, 1971), p. 834 (hereafter cited as *OSHA Legis. Hist.*).
10. The original Senate bill, S.2193, 91st Cong. 1st Sess. (1969), was introduced by Senator Harrison Williams. The Javits amendment was added during deliberations of the Senate Committee on Labor and Public Welfare. See *OSHA Legis. Hist.,* p. 242.
11. Senator Javits had originally introduced the Nixon administration's bill, S.2788, 91st Cong., 1st Sess. (1969); the quoted passage is the senator's explanation of his amendment to the original Williams bill. See Senate (S) Report no. 91–1282 (1970), p. 58; *OSHA Legis. Hist.,* p. 197.
12. Statement of Senator Dominick, *Congressional Record,* 116 (1970): 37614.
13. *OSHA Legis. Hist.,* p. 367.
14. Statement of Senator Dominick, p. 37622.
15. When the OSHA bill came up for final votes after the amendment process, it passed the House 384–5 and the Senate 83–3. Although the final version was closer to the original Williams bill than to the Nixon administration's original bill, President Nixon chose to sign the bill into law on Dec. 29, 1970. *Congressional Quarterly Almanac* (1970): 675–682.
16. OSHA selected the more protective 10 ppm standard of ANSI rather

than the 25 ppm standard adopted by the American Conference of Government Industrial Hygienists. *Fed. Reg.*, 43 (1978): 5919.

17. For example, in a letter dated Apr. 23, 1976, the United Rubber, Cork, Linoleum, and Plastic Workers of America urged the secretary of labor to issue an emergency temporary standard for benzene. Secretary of Labor William J. Usery denied the request on May 18, 1976, citing a lack of scientific evidence to warrant the action. See also *Fed. Reg.*, 43 (1978): 5919.

18. See Committee on Toxicology, *Health Effects of Benzene: A Review* (Washington, D.C.: National Academy Press, 1976); and National Institute for Occupational Safety and Health [NIOSH], *Occupational Exposure to Benzene* (Washington, D.C.: U.S. Government Printing Office, 1974).

19. NIOSH recommended an emergency 1 ppm standard by letter on Oct. 27, 1976. See *Fed. Reg.*, 43 (1978): 5919.

20. For example, a report by the General Accounting Office to the House Committee on Governmental Operations had criticized the Ford administration's neglect of health hazards in the workplace. See *Performance of the Occupational Safety and Health Administration*, Hearings before the Subcommittee on Manpower and Housing, Committee on Governmental Operations, 95th Cong., 1st Sess., U.S. House of Representatives (U.S. Government Printing Office, 1977).

21. *Occupational Safety and Health Reporter*, Bureau of National Affairs (BNA), 6 (1977): 1587 (Bingham announces intention to focus regulatory efforts on health risks from toxic chemicals).

22. The ensuing account of Bingham's role in the benzene rulemaking is based in part on a personal communication by Grover Wrenn, former director of health standards at OSHA, Mar. 26, 1984, in Boston.

23. Thomas R. Bartman, "Regulating Benzene," in *Quantitative Risk Assessment in Regulation*, ed. Lester B. Lave (Washington, D.C.: Brookings Institution, 1982), p. 102.

24. *U.S. Code*, 29: 655(c).

25. The preliminary results of Infante's study were used to support the ETS for benzene. See P. F. Infante, R. A. Rinsky, J. K. Wagoner, and R. J. Young, "Leukemia in Benzene Workers," *Lancet*, July 9, 1977, pp. 76–78.

26. *Fed. Reg.*, 42 (1977): 22516.

27. *U.S. Code*, 29: 655(f).

28. The preceding two paragraphs are based on the written opinions of the justices in Industrial Union Dept., AFL-CIO v. Bingham, 570 F.2d (D.C. Cir. 1977), p. 965.

29. R. Shep Melnick, *Regulation and the Courts: The Case of the Clean Air Act* (Washington, D.C.: Brookings Institution, 1983), pp. 56, 70; and Baird, "IUD v. API," pp. 643–652.

30. James H. Jandl, "Hematologic Disorders," in *Occupational Health: Recognizing and Preventing Work-Related Disease*, ed. Barry S. Levy and David H. Wegman (Boston: Little Brown, 1983), pp. 367–371.

31. In 1977 Wilson's risk assessment was the only such analysis available for benzene. Richard Wilson, Testimony at OSHA Hearings on Proposed Standard for Occupational Exposure to Benzene, Docket H-059, U.S. Dept. of Labor, Washington, D.C., 1977, mimeo.

32. OSHA was criticized for not using CEA or CBA by Harvard economist Richard Zeckhauser. Testimony at OSHA Hearings on Proposed Standard for Occupational Exposure to Benzene.

33. Occupational Safety and Health Administration, *Economic Impact Statement: Benzene* (Washington, D.C.: U.S. Department of Labor, 1977), 2 vols.

34. One labor union proposed a 0.5 ppm PEL for oil refineries and a 1 ppm ceiling (rather than a TWA) for all other industries. Another union proposed a 1 ppm ceiling for all industries.

35. One of OSHA's major regulatory initiatives under Bingham was a proposed generic carcinogen policy designed to accelerate OSHA rulemaking on carcinogenic chemicals. *Fed. Reg.*, 42 (1977): 54148.

36. American Petroleum Institute v. OSHA, 581 F.2d (5th Cir., 1978), pp. 493, 503.

37. Industrial Union Dept. v. American Petroleum Inst., 448 U.S. Sup. Ct. (1980), p. 607 (hereafter cited as IUD v API).

38. The progression of the cotton-dust case in the federal courts was quite different. OSHA's standard was originally upheld in the D.C. Circuit in spite of challenges by both industry and labor groups. AFL-CIO v. Marshall, 199 U.S. App. D.C., 617 F.2d (1979), p. 636. On appeal the U.S. Supreme Court affirmed the D.C. Circuit's holding. American Textile Mfrs. Inst. v. Donovan, 452 U.S. (1981), p. 490 (hereafter cited as ATMI v. Donovan).

39. *Fed. Reg.*, 48 (1983): 31412–31414.

40. For journalistic coverage of the negotiations, see "Industry, Labor Continue Mediation; API Declines to Participate in Talks," *Occupational Safety and Health Reporter* (BNA), Dec. 12, 1983, pp. 797–798; and "Participants in Benzene Mediation Unable to Agree on Joint Recommendation, " *Occupational Safety and Health Reporter* (BNA), Feb. 16, 1984, pp. 989–999. For a more thorough analysis of the origins and dynamics of the benzene negotiations, see Henry H. Perritt, Jr., "Analysis of Four Negotiated Rulemaking Efforts," in *Final Report to the Administrative Conference of the United States*, (New York: American Bar Association, 1985), pp. 64–128.

41. United Steelworkers of America v. Donovan, Case no. 84–5842, D.C. Circuit Court of Appeals, filed Dec. 10, 1984. See also "API Files Motion to Intervene as Respondent in Benzene Suit," *Occupational Safety and Health Reporter* (BNA), Jan. 17, 1985, p. 605.

42. "Doctor Cites Benzene Exposure as Likely Cause of High Cancer Death Rate at Shell Refinery," *Wall Street Journal*, Feb. 27, 1985, p. 26.

43. "Benzene Exposure at Approved Level Linked to Cancer," *Wall Street Journal*, Feb. 27, 1985, p. 26.

44. "OSHA Benzene Standard Should Range from Five to One PPM, Chemical Groups Assert," *Occupational Safety and Health Reporter* (BNA), Mar. 14, 1985, p. 779.

45. "Draft Proposal under OMB Review Would Set One PPM Limit, Five PPM Ceiling," *Occupational Safety and Health Reporter* (BNA), Apr. 4, 1985, pp. 835–836.

46. *U.S. Code*, 42: 7412 (1982).

47. *Fed. Reg.*, 46 (1977): 29332–29333.

48. *U.S. Code*, 42: 74112 (1982).

49. See John D. Graham, "The Failure of Agency-Forcing: The Regulation of Airborne Carcinogens under Section 112 of the Clean Air Act," *Duke Law Journal*, 85 (1985): 100–152.

50. *Fed. Reg.*, 46 (1977): 29333.

51. EPA, "Interim Procedures and Guidelines for Health Risk and Economic Impact Assessments of Suspected Carcinogens," *Fed. Reg.*, 41 (1976): 21402–21405.

52. *Fed. Reg.*, 46 (1977): 29332–29333.

53. *Fed. Reg.*, 45 (1980): 26660–26683.

54. *Fed. Reg.*, 45 (1980): 83448–83463; *Fed. Reg.*, 45 (1980): 83952–83967; *Fed. Reg.*, 46 (1981): 1165–1191.

55. Telephone interview with Alan Jones of EPA, Mar. 4, 1984.

56. "Two Groups Sue to Force Promulgation of Standards under Air Act by September," *Chemical Regulation Reporter* (BNA), July 22, 1983, p. 556.

57. NRDC and EDF v. EPA and William Ruckelshaus, U.S. District Court of the District of Columbia, Case no. 83–2011.

58. Telephone interview with Alan Jones, EPA, Mar. 14, 1984.

59. *Fed. Reg.*, 49 (1984): 8386.

60. "Standards on Fugitive Benzene Sources Set; EPA Proposes to Regulate Coke Oven Emissions," *Environment Reporter* (BNA), June 1, 1984, p. 61.

61. NRDC v. EPA and Ruckelshaus, Jan. 27, 1984.

62. *Fed. Reg.*, 49 (1984): 23478, 23498, 23522, 23558.

63. *Fed. Reg.*, 49 (1984): 23488.

64. Ruth Ruttenberg and Eula Bingham, "A Comprehensive Carcinogen Policy as a Framework for Regulatory Activity," in *Management of Assessed Risk for Carcinogens*, ed. William J. Nicholson (New York: Annals of the New York Academy of Sciences, 1981), p. 17.

65. ATMI v. Donovan, p. 509.

66. This point was originally made by Kelman, "Occupational Safety and Health Administration," in Wilson, *Politics of Regulation*, pp. 250–251.

67. A general discussion of the link between professional ideology and bureaucratic health is available in James Q. Wilson, "The Politics of Regulation," in *The Social Responsibility of Business*, ed. James McKie (Washington, D.C.: Brookings Institution, 1973), p. 162.

68. Lester B. Lave, *The Strategy of Social Regulation* (Washington, D.C.: Brookings Institution, 1981), p. 14.

69. ATMI v. Donovan, p. 514.
70. Society of Plastics Industries v. OSHA, 508 F.2d (2nd Cir.), pp. 1301, 1309, cert. denied, 421 U.S. (1975), p. 992.
71. United Steelworkers v. Marshall, 647 F.2d (D.C. Cir. 1980), pp. 1264–1265 (hereafter cited as USW v. Marshall).
72. American Iron and Steel Institute v. OSHA, 508 F.2d (3rd Cir. 1978), cert. dismissed, 448 U.S. 917 (1980).
73. Ibid., p. 478.
74. For an excellent article supporting the feasibility doctrine, see Jeffrey Lewis Berger and Steven D. Riskin, "Economic and Technological Feasibility in Regulating Toxic Substances under the Occupational Safety and Health Act," *Ecology Law Quarterly*, 7 (1978): 285–358.
75. IUD v. API, p. 641.
76. Ibid., p. 664 (Chief Justice Burger, concurring). On the legal doctrine of *de minimis* risk, see Alabama Power Co. v. Costle, 204 U.S. App. D.C., pp.88–89; 636 F.2d (1979), pp. 360–361.
77. A close reading of the plurality opinion reveals that the significant-risk doctrine is motivated, at least in part, by priority-setting concerns. See IUD v. API, pp. 643–644 and 645, especially n. 49. See also John Mendeloff, "Priority Setting at OSHA: Is There Anything Out There Worth Regulating?" Paper presented at Annual Research Conference of Association of Public Policy Analysis and Management, Philadelphia, Oct. 21, 1983, pp. 1–2.
78. In fact, the plurality hints that OSHA's priority-setting procedures may be immune from judicial review, IUD v. API, p. 644, n. 49.
79. David Doniger argues that because the majority had no common rationale, no rule of law emerged from IUD v. API. See David D. Doniger, "Defeat in the Benzene Exposure Case No Death Knell for OSHA Standards," *National Law Journal*, Sept. 15, 1980, pp. 26–27. On the legal significance of plurality opinions, see "The Precedential Value of Supreme Court Plurality Decisions," *Columbia Law Review*, 80 (1980): 756–778.
80. USW v. Marshall, pp. 1189, 1245–1246, n. 84 (Judge Skelly Wright), cert. denied, 453 U.S. (1981), p. 913.
81. ATMI v. Donovan, pp. 513–514, n. 32.
82. USW. v. Marshall, p. 1248.
83. Texas Independent Ginners Ass'n v. Marshall, 630 F.2d (5th Cir. 1980), p. 398.
84. Bingham deleted provisions of the OSHA cancer policy that were perceived to be inconsistent with the significant-risk doctrine. See *Fed. Reg.*, 46 (1981): 4889. She also proposed amendments to the cancer policy to incorporate quantitative risk assessment, *Fed. Reg.*, 46 (1980): 7402, but these were subsequently withdrawn by Auchter pending a review of the entire OSHA cancer policy. See *Fed. Reg.*, 47 (1982): 1987.
85. IUD v. API, p. 655.

86. *Fed. Reg.*, 47 (1982): 15358 (proposed arsenic rule); *Fed. Reg.*, 48 (1983): 1864 (final arsenic rule); *Fed. Reg.*, 48 (1983): 51086 (proposed ETS for asbestos).

87. IUD v. API, pp. 656–657.

88. See Testimony of Representative Don Ritter in *Risk/Benefit Analysis in the Legislative Process*, Joint Hearings of House Committee on Science and Technology and Senate Committee on Commerce, 96th Cong., 1st sess., July 24–25, 1979, pp. 113–118.

89. Harvey Brooks, personal communication, June 14, 1984.

90. *Fed. Reg.*, 48 (1983): 1864–1866.

91. *Fed. Reg.*, 48 (1983): 31413 (summarizes benzene risk assessments). For example, see Mary C. White, Peter F. Infante, and Kenneth C. Chu, "A Quantitative Estimate of Leukemia Mortality Associated with Occupational Exposure to Benzene," *Risk Analysis*, 2 (1982): 195–204.

92. A plurality of the Supreme Court was clearly impressed with Wilson's assessment. IUD v. API, pp. 635, 654–655.

93. See Edmund C. Crouch and Richard Wilson, *Risk/Benefit Analysis* (Cambridge, Mass.: Ballinger, 1982), pp. 178–179 and 198–199.

94. This point was raised by the United Steelworkers (USW) in a recent OSHA rulemaking. See *Fed. Reg.*, 48 (1983): 1902 (summary of USW statement).

95. A large literature in economics exists on this topic. See, for example, W. Kip Viscusi, *Employment Hazards: An Investigation of Market Performance* (Cambridge, Mass.: Harvard University Press, 1979).

96. Testimony of Richard Zeckhauser, OSHA's Proposed Generic Cancer Policy, U.S. Dept. of Labor, 1978, p. 13, mimeo.

97. For an extensive statement of this position, see Robert S. Smith, *The Occupational Safety and Health Act* (Washington, D.C.: American Enterprise Institute, 1976).

98. The quotation is reprinted in *Fed. Reg.*, 45 (1980): 5249. See generally, Nicholas A. Ashford, "Alternatives to Cost-Benefit Analysis in Regulatory Decision Making," in Nicholson, *Management of Assessed Risk for Carcinogens*, pp. 129–138.

99. Robert W. Crandall, "The Use of Cost-Benefit Analysis in Regulatory Decision Making," in Nicholson, *Management of Assessed Risk for Carcinogens*, p. 105.

100. ATMI v. Donovan, p. 509.

101. See both IUD v. API, pp. 643–644; and ATMI v. Donovan, p. 509, n. 29.

102. See, for example, "Regulatory Reform Bill Dead in Lame Duck," *National Journal*, 15 (1983): 105.

103. On the role of the executive order, see Judith D. Bentkover, "The Role of Benefits Assessment in Public Policy Development," in *Benefits Assessment: The State of the Art*, ed. J. D. Bentkover (Boston: D. Reidel Publishing, 1986), pp. 1–4.

104. IUD v. API, p. 646 (Justice Powell); pp. 655–666 (Justice Stevens).

105. Decision analysis offers approaches for converting scientific uncertainty

into subjective probabilities. These probabilities can then be used to make probabilistic net-benefit estimates for regulatory alternatives. See, generally, Howard Raiffa, *Decision Analysis: Introductory Lectures on Choices under Uncertainty* (Reading, Mass.: Addison Wesley, 1968).

106. John Mendeloff, "Does Overregulation Cause Underregulation?" *Regulation* (Sept./Oct. 1981): 48.

107. W. Kip Viscusi, *Risk by Choice* (Cambridge, Mass.: Harvard University Press, 1983), p. 14.

108. "Ruckelshaus: Give the Policy Makers More Flexibility," *National Journal*, Dec. 3, 1983, 2530 (interview with Ruckelshaus).

109. IUD v. API, p. 672 (Justice Rehnquist concurring in judgment).

110. For analysis of the significant-risk doctrine, see Peter F. Stone, "The Significant-Risk Requirement in OSHA Regulation of Carcinogens: IUD v. API," *Stanford Law Review*, 33 (1981): 564.

■ 5. Interpreting the Scientfic Evidence on Benzene and Cancer

1. Donald Hunter, *The Diseases of Occupations*, 5th ed. (London: English Universities Press, 1975), pp. 471–485.

2. James H. Jandl, "Hematologic Disorders," in *Occupational Health: Recognizing and Preventing Work-Related Disease*, ed. B. S. Levy and D. H. Wegman (Boston: Little, Brown, 1983), pp. 357–371.

3. C. G. Santensson,"Uber Chronische Vergiftung mit Steinkohlentheerbenzin: Vir Todesfalle," *Archives fuer Hygiene Berlin*, 31 (1897): 336.

4. L. Selling, "Benzol as a Leucotoxin: Studies on the Degeneration and Regeneration of the Blood and Hematopoietic Organs," *Bulletin of Johns Hopkins Hospital*, 17 (1916): 83–142; L. Selling, "A Preliminary Report of Some Cases of Purpura Haemorrhagica due to Benzol Poisoning," *Bulletin of Johns Hopkins Hospital*, 21 (1910): 33–37; C. R. Newton, "Industrial Blood Poisons," *Journal of the American Medical Association*, 74 (1920): 1149.

5. A. Hamilton, "The Growing Menace of Benzene (Benzol) Poisoning in American Industry," *Journal of the American Medical Association*, 78 (1922): 627–630.

6. P. Delore and C. Borgomano, "Acute Leukemia Following Benzene Poisoning: On the Toxic Origin of Certain Acute Leukaemias and the Relation to Serious Anaemias," *Journal de Médecine de Lyon*, 9 (1928): 227–233.

7. F. Penati and E. C. Vigliani, "Sui Problema delle Mielopatie Aplastiche, Pseudo-aplastiche e Leucemiche du Benzolo," *Rassegna di Medicina Industriale*, 9 (1938): 345–361.

8. T. B. Mallory, E. A. Gall, and W. J. Brickley, "Chronic Exposure to Benzene (Benzol), III: The Pathologic Results," *Journal of Industrial Hygiene and Toxicology*, 21 (1939): 355–377.

9. Enrico C. Vigliani and Giulio Saita, "Benzene and Leukemia," *New England*

Journal of Medicine, 271, no. 17 (1964): 872–876. E. C. Vigliani and A. Forni, "Benzene and Leukemia," *Environmental Research,* 19 (1976): 122–127."

10. Vigliani and Forni, "Benzene and Leukemia," p. 126.

11. M. Aksoy, "Leukemia in Workers Due to Occupational Exposure to Benzene," *New Istanbul Contributions to Clinical Science,* 12 (1977): 3–14, esp. 4.

12. M. Aksoy, "Different Types of Malignancies due to Occupational Exposure to Benzene: A Review of Recent Observations in Turkey," *Environmental Research,* 23 (1980): 181–190.

13. International Agency for Research on Cancer [IARC], *Monographs on the Evaluation of Carcinogenic Risk of Chemicals to Humans,* vol. 29, *Some Industrial Chemicals and Dyestuffs* (Geneva: World Health Organization, 1982), 92–148.

14. B. Goldstein, Presentation at Collegium Ramazzini Meeting on Benzene, New York City, Nov. 3–4, 1983.

15. A. Forni and E. C. Vigliani, "Chemical Leukemogenesis in Man," *Series in Haematology,* 7 (1974): 211–223.

16. Community Working Group, "Establishment of Mak-Werte, Senate Committee for the Examination of Hazardous Industrial Materials," in *Benzene in the Work Environment: Considerations Bearing on the Question of Safe Concentrations of Benzene in the Work Environment,* unpublished, 1974.

17. Vigliani and Saita, "Benzene and Leukemia," p. 875.

18. Testimony of Muzaffer Aksoy, M.D., to Occupational Safety and Health Administration, U.S. Department of Labor, July 13, 1977.

19. Testimony of Richard Wilson at OSHA Hearing on Proposed Standard for Occupational Exposure to Benzene, Docket no. H-059, 1977.

20. Carcinogen Assessment Group [CAG], *Final Report on Population Risk to Ambient Benzene Exposures* (Washington, D.C.: U.S. Environmental Protection Agency, 1979).

21. O. Wong, "An Industry-wide Mortality Study of Chemical Workers Occupationally Exposed to Benzene," unpublished report submitted to Chemical Manufacturers Association, 1983).

22. The following wrote reviews (unpublished, 1983) of Wong's study of chemical workers: P. Enterline, A. M. Lilienfeld, B. MacMahon, and H. E. Rockette.

23. P. F. Infante, R. A. Rinsky, J. K. Wagoner, and R. J. Young, "Leukemia in Benzene Workers," *Lancet,* July 9, 1977, pp. 76–78.

24. R. A. Rinsky, F. J. Young, and A. B. Smith, "Leukemia in Benzene Workers," *American Journal of Industrial Medicine,* 2 (1981): 217–245.

25. Infante et al., "Leukemia in Benzene Workers," p. 76.

26. P. F. Infante, R. A. Rinsky, J. K. Wagoner, R. J. Young, Letter to the Editor, *Lancet,* Oct. 22, 1977, pp. 868–869.

27. Infante et al., "Leukemia in Benzene Workers," p. 76.

28. Ibid., p. 78.

29. I. R. Tabershaw and S. H. Lamm, "Benzene and Leukemia, " *Lancet*, Oct. 22, 1977, pp. 867–868.

30. Infante et al., Letter to the Editor.

31. S. H. Lamm and R. Wilson, "Risk Assessment for Low-Level Benzene Exposures: A Historical Perspective," unpublished report, Oct. 1983, p. 5.

32. Ibid., pp. 12–13.

33. J. J. Thorpe, "Epidemiologic Survey of Leukemia in Persons Potentially Exposed to Benzene," *Journal of Occupational Medicine*, 17 (1974): 5–6.

34. S. M. Brown, Letter to the Editor, "Leukemia and Potential Benzene Exposure," *Journal of Occupational Medicine*, 17 (1975): 6.

35. J. J. Thorpe, Response to Letter by S. M. Brown, *Journal of Occupational Medicine*, 17 (1975): 6.

36. Wong, "Industry-wide Mortality Study," pp. 3–4.

37. L. Rushton and M. R. Alderson, "A Case-Control Study to Investigate the Association between Exposure to Benzene and Deaths from Leukaemia in Oil Refinery Workers," *British Journal of Cancer*, 43 (1981b): 77–84, esp. 77.

38. Wong, "Industry-wide Mortality Study," pp. 66–67.

39. MacMahon, "Review of [Wong's] Draft Report," pp. 9–10.

40. G. M. Ott, J. C. Townsend, W. A. Fishback, and R. A. Langer, "Mortality among Individuals Occupationally Exposed to Benzene," *Archives of Environmental Health*, 33 (Jan./Feb. 1978): 3–10, esp. 9.

41. P. F. Infante and W. C. White, "Benzene: Epidemiologic Observations of Leukemia by Cell Type and Adverse Health Effects Associated with Low-Level Exposure," *Environmental Health Perspectives*, 52 (1983): 75–82.

42. Richard Wilson, personal communication, 1984.

43. See MacMahon, "Review of [Wong's] Draft Report," pp. 9–10; and Environmental Protection Agency, *Assessment of Health Effects of Benzene Germane to Low-Level Exposure*, EPA-600/1-78-061 (Washington, D.C.: U.S. Government Printing Office, 1978.

44. Ott et al., "Mortality among Individuals," p. 3.

45. P. Decoufle, W. A. Blattner, and A. Blair, "Mortality among Chemical Workers Exposed to Benzene and Other Agents," *Environmental Research*, 30 (1983): 16–25, esp. 16.

46. P. Cole, "Acute Myelogenous Leukemia and Other Forms of Leukemia at Wood River," report submitted to Shell Oil Company, 1985.

47. Statement of R. E. Joyner, corporate medical director, Shell Oil Co., "Employee Communication," no. 24, 1985.

48. "Doctor Cites Benzene Exposures as Likely Cause of High Cancer Death Rate at Shell Refinery," *Wall Street Journal*, Feb. 14, 1985, p. 4.

49. Letter from R. E. Joyner to Dr. J. Donald Miller, director, NIOSH, July 28, 1983, mimeo.

50. R. D. Irons, H. A. Heck, B. J. Moore, and K. A. Muirhead, "Effects of

Short Term Benzene Administration on Bone Marrow Cell Cycle Kinetics in the Rat," *Toxicology and Applied Pharmacology*, 51 (1979): 399–409.

51. R. S. Brief, J. Lynch, T. Bernath, and R. A. Scala, "Benzene in the Workplace," *American Industrial Hygiene Association Journal*, 41 (1980): 616–623.

52. H. G. S. Van Raalte, O. Grasso, and D. Irvine, "Tackling a Very Difficult Problem," *Risk Analysis*, 4 (1984): 1–2.

53. M. C. White, P. F. Infante, and K. C. Chu, "A Quantitative Estimate of Leukemia Mortality Associated with Occupational Exposure to Benzene," *Risk Analysis*, 2 (1982): 195–204.

54. Decoufle et al., "Mortality among Chemical Workers," p. 17.

55. Occupational Safety and Health Administration, "Occupational Exposure to Benzene: Permanent Standard," *Fed. Reg.*, 43 (1978): 5918–5970.

56. Occupational Safety and Health Administration, "Occupational Exposure to Benzene, Proposed Standard," transcript of public hearing, U.S. Department of Labor, Washington, D.C., July 19–Aug. 10, 1977.

57. G. Pollini and R. Colombi, "Lymphocyte Chromosome Damage in Benzene Blood Dyscrasia," *Medicina del Lavoro*, 55 (1964): 641–654; G. Pollini, E. Strosselli, and R. Colombi, "Relationship between Chromosomal Alternations and Severity of Benzol Blood Dyscrasia," ibid., pp. 735–751; I. M. Tough, and W. M. Court-Brown, "Chromosome Aberrations and Exposure to Ambient Benzene," *Lancet*, 1 (1965): 684; I. M. Tough, P. G. Smith, W. M. Court-Brown, and D. G. Hamden, "Chromosome Studies in Workers Exposed to Atmospheric Benzene: The Possible Influence of Age," *European Journal of Cancer*, 6 (1970): 49–55; A. Forni and L. Moreo, "Chromosome Studies in a Case of Benzene-induced Erythroleukaemia," *European Journal of Cancer*, 5 (1969): 459–463; A. Forni, D. Pacifico, and A. Limonta, "Chromosome Studies in Workers Exposed to Benzene or Toluene or Both," *Archives of Environmental Health*, 22 (1971): 373–378.

58. M. Kissling and B. Speck, "Chromosome Aberrations Experimental Benzene Intoxification," *Helvetica Medica Acta*, 36 (1972): 59–66.

59. Raymond R. Tice, Daniel L. Costa, and Robert T. Drew, "Cytogenetic Effects of Inhaled Benzene in Murine Bone Marrow: Induction of Sister Chromatid Exchanges, Chromosomal Aberrations and Cellular Proliferation Inhibition in DBA/2 Mice," *Proceedings of the National Academy of Sciences (USA)*, 77 (Apr. 1980): 2148–2152.

60. A. Koizumi, Y. Dobashi, Y. Tachibana, K. Tsuda, and H. Katsunuma, "Cytokinetic and Cytogenetic Changes in Cultured Human Leucocytes and HeLa Cells Induced by Benzene," *Industrial Health*, 12 (1974): 23–29; K. Morimoto, "Analysis of Combined Effects of Benzene with Radiation on Chromosomes in Cultured Human Leucocytes," *Japanese Journal of Industrial Health*, 18 (1976): 23–24.

61. G. Hartwich and G. Schwanitz, "Chromosominuntersuchungen Nach

Chronischer Benzol-Exposition," *Deutsche Medizinische Wochenschrift*, 97 (1972): 45–49.

62. B. J. Dean, "Genetic Toxicology of Benzene, Toluene, Xylenes, and Phenols," *Mutation Research*, 47 (1978): 75–97.

63. S. R. Wolman, "Cytologic and Cytogenetic Effects of Benzene," *Toxicology and Environmental Health Supplement*, 2 (1977): 63–69.

64. Tough et al., "Chromosome Studies in Workers."

65. D. Picciano, "Cytogenetic Study of Workers Exposed to Benzene," *Environmental Research*, 19 (1979): 33–38.

66. J. L. Hamerton, A. I. Taylor, R. Angell, and V. M. McGuire, "Chromosome Investigations of a Small Isolated Human Population: Chromosome Abnormalities and Distributions of Chromosome Counts, According to Age and Sex among the Population of Tristan da Cunha," *Nature*, 206 (1965): 1232–1234.

67. Picciano, "Cytogenetic Study of Workers."

68. *Fed. Reg.*, 49 (1984): 23481.

69. D. J. Kilan and R. C. Daniel, "A Cytogenetic Study of Workers Exposed to Benzene in the Texas Division of Dow Chemical, U.S.A.," unpublished report, Feb. 27, 1978.

70. B. D. Goldstein, C. A. Snyder, S. Laskin, I. Bromber, R. E. Albert, and N. Nelson, "Myelogenous Leukemia in Rodents Inhaling Benzene," *Toxicology Letters*, 13 (1982): 169–170.

71. See C. Maltoni and C. Scarnato, "First Experimental Demonstration of the Carcinogenic Effects of Benzene," *Medicina del Lavoro*, 5 (1979): 352–357; and C. Maltoni, B. Conti, and G. Cotti, "Benzene: A Multipotential Carcinogen," *American Journal of Industrial Medicine*, 4 (1983): 589–630.

72. Maltoni, Conti, and Cotti, "Benzene: A Multipotential Carcinogen."

73. James Jandl, personal communication, 1984. Also see critiques of Goldstein's results by Cesare Maltoni, "Myths and Facts in the History of Benzene Carcinogenicity," in *Carcinogenicity and Toxicity of Benzene*, ed. Myron A. Mehlman (Princeton: Princeton Scientific Publishers, 1983), p. 6.

74. Maltoni, Conti, and Cotti, "Benzene: A Multipotential Carcinogen."

75. National Toxicology Program [NTP], *Technical Report on the Toxicology and Carcinogenesis Studies of Benzene in F344/N Rats and B6C3F1 Mice* (Washington, D.C.: Department of Health and Human Services, 1983).

76. Goldstein et al., "Myelogenous Leukemia in Rodents."

77. James Jandl, personal communication.

78. J. P. Lyon, "Mutagenicity Studies with Benzene," *Dissertation Abstracts International*, 36–B (1976).

79. P. O. Nylander, H. Olfsson, B. Rasmuson, and H. Svahlin, "Mutagenic Effects of Petrol in Drosophila Melanogaster, I: Effects of Benzene and 1,2-Dichloroethane," *Mutatation Research*, 57 (1978): 163–167.

80. James Jandl, personal communication, 1984. See, generally, Jandl, "Hematologic Disorders," in Levy and Wegman, *Occupational Health*, pp. 367–371.

81. *Fed. Reg.*, 43 (1978): 5954. Richard D. Irons, personal communication, 1984.

82. Kurt S. Isselbacher, *Principles of Internal Medicine,* 9th ed. (New York: McGraw-Hill, 1980).

83. OSHA, "Occupational Exposure to Benzene," *Fed. Reg.*, 50 (1985): 50529.

84. Bernard Goldstein, personal communication, 1983.

- 6. Quantifying Cancer Risks

1. C. S. Weil, "Statistics vs. Safety Factors and Scientific Judgment in the Evaluation of Safety for Man," *Toxicology and Applied Pharmocology,* 21 (1972): 454–463.

2. See U.S. Office of Science and Technology Policy [OSTP], "Chemical Carcinogens: A Review of the Science and Its Associated Principles," *Fed. Reg.*, 50 (1985): 10438–40.

3. On the development of risk assessment at FDA, see Peter B. Hutt, "Use of Quantitative Risk Assessment in Regulatory Decisionmaking under Federal Health and Safety Statutes," in *Risk Quantitation and Regulatory Policy,* ed. D. Hoel, R. Merrill, and F. Perera (New York: Cold Spring Harbor Laboratory, 1985), pp. 15–29; on EPA see Roy E. Albert, R. E. Train, and E. Anderson, "Rationale Developed by the Environmental Protection Agency for the Assessment of Carcinogenic Risks," *Journal of the National Cancer Institute,* 58 (1977): 1537.

4. For an introductory essay on how a decision analyst approaches risk assessment, see D. Warner North, "Decision Analysis and Risk Assessment," paper presented to the Symposium on Risk Assessment, Electric Power Research Institute, Monterey, California, Aug. 1984; excerpts reprinted in "Cancer and the Problems of Risk Assessment," *Electric Power Research Institute Journal* (Dec. 1984): 26–35.

5. See, for example, Howard Raiffa, *Decision Analysis: Introductory Lectures on Choices under Uncertainty* (Reading, Mass.: Addison-Wesley, 1970); R. Howard and J. Matheson, eds., *Readings on the Principles and Applications of Decision Analysis* (Menlo Park, Calif.: Strategic Decisions Group, 1983); R. C. Keeney and H. Raiffa, *Decisions with Multiple Objectives: Preferences and Value Tradeoffs* (New York: John Wiley and Sons, 1976).

6. For discussion of these models, see OSTP, "Chemical Carcinogens," pp. 10438–10440.

7. See P. Armitage and R. Doll, "Stochastic Models for Carcinogenesis," in *Proceedings of the Fourth Berkeley Symposium on Mathematics, Statistics and Probability,* vol. 4, ed. L. Lecam and J. Weyman (Berkeley: University of California Press, 1961), pp. 19–38.

8. See, for example, K. S. Crump, "Mechanisms Leading to Dose-Response Models," in *Principles of Health Risk Assessment,* ed. Paolo Ricci (Englewood Cliffs, N.J.: Prentice-Hall, 1984), pp. 187–227.

9. D. M. Siegel, V. H. Frankos, and M. S. Schneiderman, "Formaldehyde Risk Assessment for Occupationally Exposed Workers," *Regulatory Toxicology and Pharmacology* 3 (1983): 355–371.

10. OSHA, "Occupational Exposure to Formaldehyde," *Fed. Reg.*, 50 (1985): 50458. See also Robert L. Sielken, Jr., "A Quantitative Look at the Low Dose Cancer Risk in Rats Due to Formaldehyde Inhalation," unpublished paper, Texas A and M University, Jan. 1984.

11. OSHA, "Occupational Exposure to Formaldehyde," p. 50452.

12. For EPA's view, see "Proposed Guidelines for Carcinogen Risk Assessment," *Fed. Reg.*, 49 (1984): 46298.

13. Ibid.; see also EPA, "Formaldehyde: Determination of Significant Risk" *Fed. Reg.*, 49 (May 23, 1984): 21886; U.S. Consumer Product Safety Commission [CPSC], "Ban of Urea-Formaldehyde Foam Insulation," *Fed. Reg.*, 47 (1982): 14372.

14. See E. C. Anderson and the Carcinogen Assessment Group, "Quantitative Approaches in Use to Assess Cancer Risk," *Risk Analysis*, 3 (1983): 277–295.

15. Testimony of Kenneth Crump, reprinted in OSHA, "Occupational Exposure to Formaldehyde," p. 50452.

16. Comment of Robert L. Sielken, Jr., to OSHA, Dec. 6, 1984, mimeo, pp. 9–10.

17. EPA, "Formaldehyde: Determination of Significant Risk," pp. 21887–21890.

18. OSHA, "Occupational Exposure to Benzene," p. 50535.

19. See D. Krewski and J. Van Ryzin, "Dose Response Models for Quantal Response Toxicity Data," in *Statistics and Related Topics*, ed. D. Csorgo, R. Dawson, and E. Salch (Amsterdam: North Holland, 1981), pp. 201–203.

20. Kenny S. Crump and Bruce C. Allen, "Quantitative Estimates of Risk from Occupational Exposure to Benzene," unpublished report to OSHA, May 1984, p. 24. An exception was a benzene risk assessment by Crump and Allen, yet even there the relative-risk model was preferred to the absolute-risk model on intuitive grounds.

21. Testimony of Richard Wilson on OSHA's Proposed Benzene Standard, 1977, mimeo.

22. Brian MacMahon, "Formal Comment Submitted to OSHA on Benzene Risk Assessment," 1983, mimeo.

23. IARC, *Monographs on the Evaluation of Carcinogenic Risk of Chemicals to Humans*, vol. 29, *Some Industrial Chemicals and Dyestuffs* (Geneva: World Health Organization, 1982), 397.

24. Marjorie Sun, "Risk Estimate Vanishes from Benzene Report," *Science*, 212 (1982): 914–915.

25. Muzaffer Aksoy, "Leukemia in Workers Due to Occupational Exposure to Benzene," *New Istanbul Contribution to Clinical Science*, 12, no. 3 (1977): 5.

26. Carcinogen Assessment Group, *Final Report on Population Risk to Ambient Benzene Exposure* (Washington, D.C.: Environmental Protection Agency, 1979).

27. Richard Wilson, personal communication, 1984.

28. Carcinogen Assessment Group, *Interim Quantitative Cancer Unit Risk Estimates Due to Inhalation of Benzene* (Washington, D.C.: Environmental Protection Agency, Feb. 15, 1985).

29. Richard Wilson, personal communication, 1985.

30. M. C. White, P. F. Infante, and K. C. Chu, "A Quantitative Estimate of Leukemia Mortality Associated with Occupational Exposure to Benzene," *Risk Analysis,* 2 (1982): 195–204.

31. Philip Cole, personal communication, 1984.

32. See California Department of Health Services [DHS], *Report to the Scientific Review Panel on Benzene* (Sacramento: California DHS, Nov. 27, 1984); EPA, "NESHPs; Regulation of Benzene," *Fed. Reg.,* 49 (1984): 23478.

33. California DHS, *Report,* pp. 51, 56.

34. EPA, "Proposed Guidelines for Carcinogen Risk Assessment," p. 46298.

35. California DHS, *Report,* p. 4.

36. OSHA, "Occupational Exposure to Formaldehyde," p. 50449.

37. See R. A. Squire and L. L. Cameron, "An Analysis of Potential Carcinogenic Risk from Formaldehyde," *Regulatory Toxicology and Pharmacology,* 4 (1984): 107–129.

38. OSHA, "Occupational Exposure to Formaldehyde," p. 50455.

39. Consensus Conference on Formaldehyde, "Report on the Consensus Conference on Formaldehyde," *Environmental Health Perspectives,* 58 (1984): 356.

40. EPA, "Proposed Guidelines for Carcinogen Risk Assessment," p. 46298.

41. OSHA, "Occupational Exposure to Formaldehyde," p. 50450.

42. Ibid.

43. Ibid.

44. Consensus Conference on Formaldehyde, "Report," p. 355.

45. EPA, "Proposed Guidelines for Carcinogen Risk Assessment," p. 46298.

46. Ibid., p. 46298.

47. California DHS, *Report,* p. 6.

48. Under contract to EPA, Crump has developed the multistage model for easy application. See K. S. Crump and R. B. Howe, *Approaches to Carcinogenic, Mutagenic and Teratogenic Risk Assessment,* Final Report to U.S. EPA, contract no. 68-01-5975, Task A, Subtask, 5, Summary Report, 1980; See also R. B. Howe and K. S. Crump, "A Computer Program to Extrapolate Quantal Animal Toxicity Data to Low Doses," report to OSHA, contract no. 41 USL 252 C3, 1983. Crump was also a member of a key NAS panel (see Chapter 7) that recommended uniform risk assessment guidelines.

49. Crump and Allen, "Quantitative Estimates," p. 29.
50. EPA, "Proposed Guidelines for Carcinogen Risk Assessment," p. 46299.
51. See C. Maltoni and G. Lefemine, "Carcinogenicity Assays to Vinyl Chloride: Current Results," *Annals of the New York Academy of Sciences*, 246 (1975): 195–224.
52. EPA, "Formaldehyde: Determination of Significant Risk," p. 21880.
53. D. Hattis, G. Mitchell, J. McCleary-Jones, and N. Gorelick, *Control of Occupational Exposures to Formaldehyde: A Case Study of Methodology for Assessing the Health and Economic Impacts of OSHA Health Standards* unpublished report, MIT Center for Policy Alternatives, Cambridge, Mass., 1981.
54. Crump and Allen, "Quantitative Estimates," p. 21.
55. T. B. Starr and R. D. Buck, "The Importance of Delivered Dose in Estimating Low-Dose Cancer Risk From Inhalation Exposure to Formaldehyde," *Fundamental Applied Toxicology*, 4 (1984): 740–753.
56. OSHA, "Occupational Exposure to Formaldehyde," p. 50453.
57. Paxton and others quoted, ibid., p. 50453.

- 7. Science and Policy Conflict

1. Office of Technology Assessment, *Technologies for Determining Cancer Risks from the Environment* (Washington, D.C.: U.S. Government Printing Office, 1981), pp. 113–152.
2. Ibid.
3. The following papers provide a useful start in learning this literature: K. S. Crump, D. G. Hoel, C. H. Langley, and R. Peto, "Fundamental Carcinogenic Processes and Their Implication for Low Dose Risk Assessment," *Cancer Research*, 36 (1976): 2973–2979; J. Cornfield, "Carcinogenic Risk Assessment," *Science*, 198 (1977): 691–699; H. O. Hartley and R. L. Sielken, "Estimation of 'Safe Doses' in Carcinogenic Experiments," *Biometrics*, 33 (1977): 1–30; E. Crouch and R. Wilson, "Interspecies Comparison of Carcinogenic Potency," *Journal of Toxicology and Environmental Health*, 5 (1978): 1095–1118; D. W. Gaylor and R. L. Kodell, "Linear Interpolation Algorithm for Low Dose Risk Assessment of Toxic Substances," *Journal of Environmental Pathology Toxicology*, 4 (1980): 305–312; Alice S. Whittemore, "Mathematical Models of Cancer and Their Use in Risk Assessment," *Journal of Environmental Pathology and Toxicology*, 3 (1980): 352–362; and D. G. Hoel, N. L. Kaplan, and M. L. Anderson, "The Implication of Nonlinear Kinetics on Risk Estimation in Carcinogenesis," *Science*, 219 (1983): 1032–1037.
4. On the Delaney Amendment, see Richard A. Merrill and Peter Barton Hutt, *Food and Drug Law* (Mineola, N.Y.: Foundation Press, 1980); and

Peter Barton Hutt, "Use of Quantitative Risk Assessment in Regulatory Decisionmaking under Federal Health and Safety Statutes," in *Risk Quantification and Regulatory Policy*, ed. D. Hoel, R. Merrill, and F. Perera (New York: Cold Spring Harbor Laboratory, 1985), pp. 15–29.

5. John D. Graham, "The Failure of Agency-Forcing: The Regulation of Airborne Carcinogens under Section 112 of the Clean Air Act," *Duke Law Journal*, 85 (Feb. 1985): 100–150.

6. For a readable discussion of the threshold question about carcinogenesis, see Thomas H. Maugh, II, "Chemical Carcinogens: How Dangerous Are Low Doses?" *Science*, 202 (1978): 37–41.

7. On the asymmetry in costs associated with false-negative and false-positive errors, see Talbot Page, "A Generic View of Toxic Chemicals and Similar Risks," *Ecology Law Quarterly*, 7 (1978): 219–220, 230–239.

8. John C. Bailar, III, and Elaine M. Smith, "Progress against Cancer?" *New England Journal of Medicine*, May 8, 1986, pp. 1226–1232.

9. E. L. Anderson and Carcinogen Assessment Group, "Quantitative Approaches in Use to Assess Cancer Risk," *Risk Analysis*, 3 (1983): 277–295; Environmental Protection Agency, "Proposed Guidelines for Carcinogen Risk Assessment," *Fed. Reg.*, 49 (1984): 46294–46301; and Roy E. Albert, R. E. Train, and E. Anderson, "Rationale Developed by the Environmental Protection Agency for the Assessment of Carcinogenic Risks," *Journal of the National Cancer Institute*, 58 (1977): 1537.

10. An important issue that we do not address here is what measure of central tendency ("best guess") should be reported to regulators. Possibilities include the median, the mode, and the expected value of the judgmental probability distribution. In the final analysis, we believe this choice should be specified by the regulator. A more extensive rationale for best estimates of risk is articulated by Lester B. Lave, *Quantitative Risk Assessment* (Washington, D.C.: Brookings Institute, 1983).

11. As a useful starting point, see M. Granger Morgan, Max Henrion, and Samuel C. Morris, *Expert Judgments in Policy Analysis* (Upton, N.Y.: Brookhaven National Laboratory, 1980).

12. See, for example, American Industrial Health Council, "Proposals to Improve Scientific Risk Assessment for Chemical Carcinogens: Dose-Response Evaluation and Characterization of Risk," AIHC Scientific Working Paper, Feb. 1985, pp. 1–58.

13. See W. Kip Viscusi, *Risk by Choice* (Cambridge, Mass.: Harvard University Press, 1983); and Albert Nichols, *Targeting Incentives for Environmental Protection* (Cambridge, Mass.: MIT Press, 1983).

14. See OSHA's generic cancer policy: OSHA, "Identification, Classification, and Regulation of Potential Occupational Carcinogens," *Fed. Reg.*, 45 (1980): 5001–5296; and Interagency Regulatory Liaison Working Group on Risk Assessment, "Scientific Bases for Identification of Potential Carcinogens and Estimation of Risks," *Fed. Reg.*, 44 (1979): 39858.

15. National Research Council, *Risk Assessment in the Federal Government: Man-

aging the Process (Washington, D.C.: National Academy of Sciences, 1983).

16. Environmental Protection Agency, "Proposed Guidelines for Carcinogen Risk Assessment," p. 33992.

17. For discussion of this point, see Albert L. Nichols and Richard J. Zeckhauser, "The Dangers of Caution: Conservatism in Assessment and the Mismanagement of Risk," discussion paper E-85-11, John F. Kennedy School of Government, Harvard University, Nov. 1985, pp. 1–55.

18. National Research Council, *Risk Assessment*, p. 77.

19. See, for example, Milton R. Wessel, *Science and Conscience* (New York: Columbia University Press, 1980), esp. chap. 7; and Milton R. Wessel, "The State of the Science Conference: A New Approach to Scientific Decision Making," *Fundamental and Applied Toxicology*, 2 (1982): 283–288.

20. See Baruch Fischhoff, Paul Slovic, and Sarah Lichtenstein, "Knowing with Certainty: The Appropriateness of Extreme Confidence," *Journal of Experimental Psychology: Human Perceptions and Performance*, 3 (Nov. 1977): 552–564; Joan E. Sieber, "Effects of Decision Importance on Ability to Generate Warranted Subjective Uncertainty," *Journal of Personality and Social Psychology*, 30 (Nov. 1974): 688–694; and, generally, Daniel Kahneman, Paul Slovic, and Amos Tversky, eds., *Judgment under Uncertainty: Heuristics and Biases* (New York: Cambridge University Press, 1981).

21. Consensus Conference on Formaldehyde, "Report on the Consensus Conference on Formaldehyde," *Environmental Health Perspectives*, 58 (Dec. 1984): 323–381.

22. Joel Yellin, "Science, Technology, and Administrative Government: Institutional Designs for Environmental Decision Making," *Yale Law Journal*, 92 (1983): 1300–1333.

23. It might be possible to enhance the technical capabilities of the federal courts through institutional reform. See Joel Yellin, "High Technology and the Courts: Nuclear Power and the Need for Institutional Reform," *Harvard Law Review*, 94 (Jan. 1981): 489–560.

24. On the limits of judicial review of these kinds of issues, see David L. Bazelon, "Risk and Responsibility," *Science*, 205 (1979): 277–280; Patricia Wald, "Judicial Review of Complex Administrative Agency Decisions," *Annals of the American Academy for Political and Social Sciences*, 462 (July 1982): 72–86; Sheila Jasanoff and Dorothy Nelkin, "Science, Technology, and the Limits of Judicial Competence," *Science*, 204 (1981): 1211–1215; and Thomas O. McGarity, "Judicial Review of Scientific Rulemaking," *Science, Technology, and Human Values*, 9 (Winter 1984): 97–106.

25. P. J. Harter, "Negotiating Regulations: A Cure for Malaise?" *Georgetown Law Journal*, 71 (1981): 1; Lawrence S. Bacow, *Bargaining for Job Safety and Health* (Cambridge, Mass.: MIT Press, 1980); and Lawrence Susskind, "Environmental Mediation and the Accountability Problem," *Vermont Law Review*, 6 (Spring 1983): 1–47.

26. Marc J. Roberts, Stephen R. Thomas, and Michael J. Dowling, "Mapping

Scientific Disputes That Affect Public Policy Making," *Science, Technology, and Human Values*, 9 (Winter 1984): 112–122.

27. In defense of separation, see Howard Raiffa, "Science and Policy: Their Separation and Integration in Risk Analysis," in *The Risk Analysis Controversy: An Institutional Perspective*, ed. H. C. Kunreuther and E. V. Levy (New York: Springer-Verlag, 1982), p. 35. On the role of values in science, see, generally, William W. Lowrance, *Modern Science and Human Values* (New York: Oxford University Press, 1985), pp. 3–22; and Helen Longino, "Beyond 'Bad Science': Skeptical Reflections on the Value-Freedom of Scientific Inquiry," *Science, Technology and Human Values*, 8 (Winter 1983): 7–17.

28. For a similar view, see the following published speeches of former EPA Administrator William Ruckelshaus: "Science, Risk, and Public Policy," *Science*, 221 (1983): 1026–1028; and "Risk, Science, and Democracy," *Issues in Science and Technology (NAS)*, 1, no. 3 (1985): 19–38.

▪ INDEX